Placental and fetal Doppler

Diploma in Fetal Medicine Series

Series Editor: K. H. Nicolaides

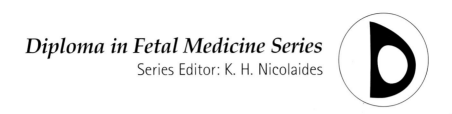

Placental and fetal Doppler

Kypros H. Nicolaides,
Giuseppe Rizzo & Kurt Hecher

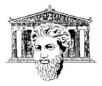

The Parthenon Publishing Group

International Publishers in Medicine, Science & Technology

NEW YORK   LONDON

Library of Congress Cataloging-in-Publication Data
Data available on request

British Library Cataloguing in Publication Data
Data available on request

ISBN 1-85070-757-X
ISSN 1467-2162

Published in the USA by
The Parthenon Publishing Group Inc.
One Blue Hill Plaza
Pearl River
New York 10965, USA

Published in the UK and Europe by
The Parthenon Publishing Group Ltd.
Casterton Hall, Carnforth
Lancs. LA6 2LA, UK

Typeset by AMA DataSet Ltd., Preston, UK
Printed and bound by Butler & Tanner Ltd., Frome and London, UK

Contents

ACKNOWLEDGEMENTS

The authors gratefully acknowledge the invaluable contributions of Simona Cicero, Nikos Kametas, Christoph Lees, Adolfo Liao and Aris Papageorgiou of the Harris Birthright Research Centre for Fetal Medicine.

Introduction

Doppler assessment of the placental circulation plays an important role in screening for impaired placentation and its complications of pre-eclampsia, intrauterine growth restriction and perinatal death. Assessment of the fetal circulation is essential in the better understanding of the pathophysiology of a wide range of pathological pregnancies and their clinical management. This book provides a comprehensive account of Doppler ultrasound in Obstetrics and will be of value to those involved in antenatal care and fetal medicine.

The first chapter explains how the competent use of Doppler ultrasound techniques requires an understanding of the hemodynamics within vessels, the capabilities and limitations of Doppler ultrasound, and the different parameters which contribute to the flow display. Chapter 2 examines how ultrasound can cause thermal and mechanical effects in the body and emphasizes the responsibility of sonographers in ensuring that ultrasound is used safely. Chapter 3 describes the methodology for obtaining and analyzing flow velocity waveforms from the uterine and umbilical arteries and fetal heart, arteries and veins and explains the physiological changes that occur during pregnancy. Chapter 4 reviews the effects of impaired placental perfusion on fetal oxygenation and the hemodynamic responses to fetal hypoxemia. Chapter 5 summarizes the results of screening studies involving assessment of impedance to flow in the uterine arteries in identifying pregnancies at risk of the complications of impaired placentation, and examines the value of prophylactic treatment with low-dose aspirin, vitamins C and E and nitric oxide donors in reducing the risk for subsequent development of pre-eclampsia. The hemodynamic responses to fetal anemia and the value of Doppler ultrasound in the management of red cell isoimmunized pregnancies are described in Chapter 6. Chapter 7 outlines the relation between impedance to flow in the uterine and umbilical arteries and maternal glycemic control or maternal nephropathy and vasculopathy in diabetes mellitus. It also describes the hemodynamic consequences of fetal acidemia and hypertrophic cardiomyopathy. Chapter 8 discusses the potential value of Doppler ultrasound in the management of pregnancies with preterm prelabor amniorrhexis, both in terms of distinction between infected and non-infected cases and in the prediction of pulmonary hypoplasia. The value of uterine and umbilical artery Doppler in identifying pregnancies at risk of pre-eclampsia, intrauterine growth restriction and perinatal death in systemic lupus erythematosus and antiphospholipid syndrome is summarized in Chapter 9. Chapter 10 reviews the Doppler findings in the placental and fetal circulations in post-term pregnancies and examines the value of Doppler in the prediction of perinatal death. Chapter 11 presents the Doppler findings in twin pregnancies and the hemodynamic changes associated with discordant fetal growth due to placental insufficiency and twin-to-twin transfusion syndrome. Chapters 12 and 13 describe the application of color Doppler in the diagnosis of cardiac and extracardiac abnormalities, respectively.

As with the introduction of any new technology into routine clinical practice, it is essential that those undertaking Doppler assessment of the placental and fetal circulations are adequately trained and their results are subjected to rigorous audit. The Fetal Medicine Foundation, under the auspices of the International Society of Ultrasound in Obstetrics and Gynecology, has introduced a process of training and certification to help to establish high standards of scanning on an international basis. The Certificates of Competence in Doppler assessment of the placental and fetal circulations are awarded to those sonographers that can perform these scans to a high standard, can demonstrate a good knowledge of the indications and limitations of Doppler and can interpret the findings in both high-risk and low-risk pregnancies.

1

Doppler ultrasound: principles and practice

Colin Deane

INTRODUCTION

In recent years, the capabilities of ultrasound flow imaging have increased enormously. Color flow imaging is now commonplace and facilities such as 'power' or 'energy' Doppler provide new ways of imaging flow. With such versatility, it is tempting to employ the technique for ever more demanding applications and to try to measure increasingly subtle changes in the maternal and fetal circulations. To avoid misinterpretation of results, however, it is essential for the user of Doppler ultrasound to be aware of the factors that affect the Doppler signal, be it a color flow image or a Doppler sonogram. Competent use of Doppler ultrasound techniques requires an understanding of three key components:

(1) The capabilities and limitations of Doppler ultrasound;

(2) The different parameters which contribute to the flow display;

(3) Blood flow in arteries and veins.

This chapter describes how these components contribute to the quality of Doppler ultrasound images. Guidelines are given on how to obtain good images in all flow imaging modes. For further reading on the subject, there are texts available covering Doppler ultrasound and blood flow theory in more detail[1–3].

BASIC PRINCIPLES

Ultrasound images of flow, whether color flow or spectral Doppler, are essentially obtained from measurements of movement. In ultrasound scanners, a series of pulses is transmitted to detect movement of blood. Echoes from stationary tissue are the same from pulse to pulse. Echoes from moving scatterers exhibit slight differences in the time for the signal to be returned to the receiver (Figure 1). These differences can be measured as a direct time difference or, more usually, in terms of a phase shift from which the 'Doppler frequency' is obtained (Figure 2). They are then processed to produce either a color flow display or a Doppler sonogram.

As can be seen from Figures 1 and 2, there has to be motion in the direction of the beam; if the flow is perpendicular to the beam, there is no relative motion from pulse to pulse. The size of the Doppler signal is dependent on:

(1) Blood velocity: as velocity increases, so does the Doppler frequency;

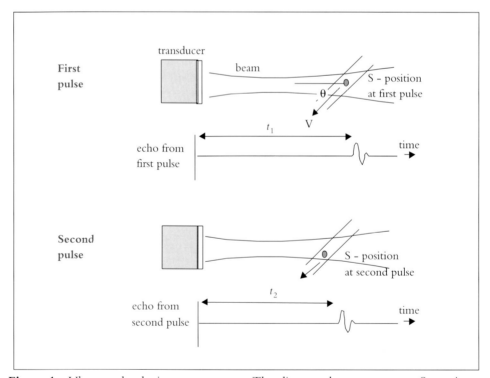

Figure 1 Ultrasound velocity measurement. The diagram shows a scatterer S moving at velocity V with a beam/flow angle θ. The velocity can be calculated by the difference in transmit-to-receive time from the first pulse to the second ($t_1 - t_2$), as the scatterer moves through the beam

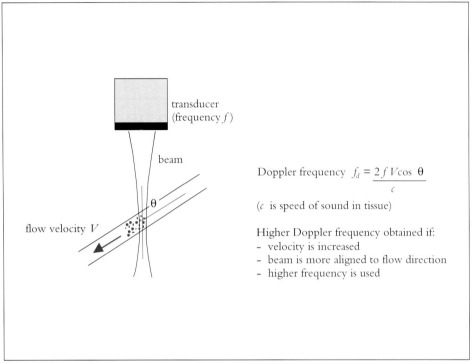

transducer
(frequency f)

beam

Doppler frequency $f_d = \dfrac{2fV\cos\theta}{c}$

(c is speed of sound in tissue)

Higher Doppler frequency obtained if:
- velocity is increased
- beam is more aligned to flow direction
- higher frequency is used

θ

flow velocity V

Figure 2 Doppler ultrasound. Doppler ultrasound measures the movement of the scatterers through the beam as a phase change in the received signal. The resulting Doppler frequency can be used to measure velocity if the beam/flow angle is known

(2) Ultrasound frequency: higher ultrasound frequencies give increased Doppler frequency. As in B-mode, lower ultrasound frequencies have better penetration. The choice of frequency is a compromise between better sensitivity to flow or better penetration;

(3) The angle of insonation: the Doppler frequency increases as the Doppler ultrasound beam becomes more aligned to the flow direction (the angle θ between the beam and the direction of flow becomes smaller). This is of the utmost importance in the use of Doppler ultrasound. The implications are illustrated schematically in Figure 3.

All types of Doppler ultrasound equipment employ filters to cut out the high-amplitude, low-frequency Doppler signals resulting from tissue movement, for instance due to vessel wall motion. Filter frequency can usually be altered by the user, for example, to exclude frequencies below 50, 100 or 200 Hz. This filter frequency limits the minimum flow velocities that can be measured.

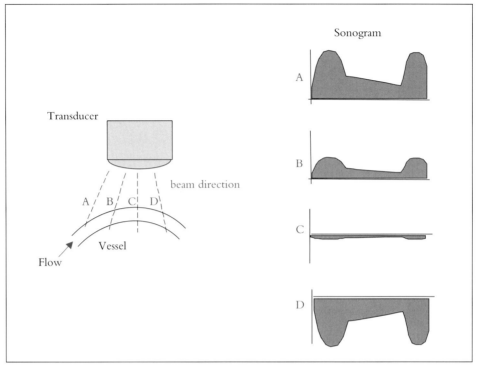

Figure 3   Effect of the Doppler angle in the sonogram. A higher-frequency Doppler signal is obtained if the beam is aligned more to the direction of flow. In the diagram, beam A is more aligned than B and produces higher-frequency Doppler signals. The beam/flow angle at C is almost 90° and there is a very poor Doppler signal. The flow at D is away from the beam and there is a negative signal

CONTINUOUS WAVE AND PULSED WAVE

As the name suggests, continuous wave systems use continuous transmission and reception of ultrasound. Doppler signals are obtained from all vessels in the path of the ultrasound beam (until the ultrasound beam becomes sufficiently attenuated due to depth). Continuous wave Doppler ultrasound is unable to determine the specific location of velocities within the beam and cannot be used to produce color flow images.

Relatively inexpensive Doppler ultrasound systems are available which employ continuous wave probes to give Doppler output without the addition of B-mode images. Continuous wave Doppler is also used in adult cardiac scanners to investigate the high velocities in the aorta.

Doppler ultrasound in general and obstetric ultrasound scanners uses pulsed wave ultrasound. This allows measurement of the depth (or range) of the flow site. Additionally, the size of the sample volume (or range gate) can be changed. Pulsed wave ultrasound is used to provide data for Doppler sonograms and color flow images.

Aliasing

Pulsed wave systems suffer from a fundamental limitation. When pulses are transmitted at a given sampling frequency (known as the pulse repetition frequency), the maximum Doppler frequency f_d that can be measured unambiguously is half the pulse repetition frequency. If the blood velocity and beam/flow angle being measured combine to give a f_d value greater than half of the pulse repetition frequency, ambiguity in the Doppler signal occurs. This ambiguity is known as aliasing. A similar effect is seen in films where wagon wheels can appear to be going backwards due to the low frame rate of the film causing misinterpretation of the movement of the wheel spokes.

The pulse repetition frequency is itself constrained by the range of the sample volume. The time interval between sampling pulses must be sufficient for a pulse to make the return journey from the transducer to the reflector and back. If a second pulse is sent before the first is received, the receiver cannot discriminate between the reflected signal from both pulses and ambiguity in the range of the sample volume ensues. As the depth of investigation increases, the journey time of the pulse to and from the reflector is increased, reducing the pulse repetition frequency for unambiguous ranging. The result is that the maximum f_d measurable decreases with depth.

Low pulse repetition frequencies are employed to examine low velocities (e.g. venous flow). The longer interval between pulses allows the scanner a better chance of identifying slow flow. Aliasing will occur if low pulse repetition frequencies or velocity scales are used and high velocities are encountered (Figure 4). Conversely, if a high pulse repetition frequency is used to examine high velocities, low velocities may not be identified.

ULTRASOUND FLOW MODES

Since color flow imaging provides a limited amount of information over a large region, and spectral Doppler provides more detailed information about a small region, the two modes are complementary and, in practice, are used as such.

Color flow imaging can be used to identify vessels requiring examination, to identify the presence and direction of flow, to highlight gross circulation anomalies

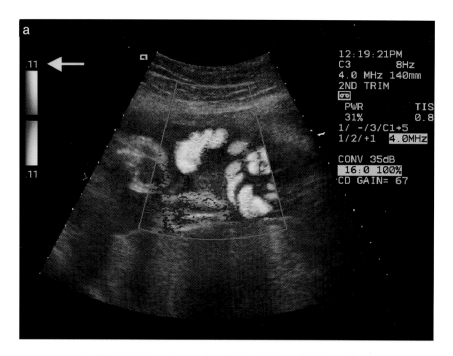

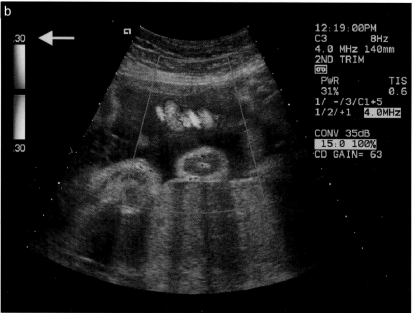

Figure 4 Color flow imaging: effects of pulse repetition frequency or scale. (a) The pulse repetition frequency or scale is set low (yellow arrow). The color image shows ambiguity within the umbilical artery and vein and there is extraneous noise. (b) The pulse repetition frequency or scale is set appropriately for the flow velocities (arrow). The color image shows the arteries and vein clearly and unambiguously

throughout the entire color flow image, and to provide beam/vessel angle correction for velocity measurements. Pulsed wave Doppler is used to provide analysis of the flow at specific sites in the vessel under investigation. When using color flow imaging with pulsed wave Doppler, the color flow/B-mode image is frozen while the pulsed wave Doppler is activated. Recently, some manufacturers have produced concurrent color flow imaging and pulsed wave Doppler, sometimes referred to as *triplex* scanning. When these modes are used simultaneously, the performance of each is decreased. Because transducer elements are employed in three modes (B-mode, color flow and pulsed wave Doppler), the frame rate is decreased, the color flow box is reduced in size and the available pulse repetition frequency is reduced, leading to increased susceptibility to aliasing.

Power Doppler is also referred to as energy Doppler, amplitude Doppler and Doppler angiography. The magnitude of the color flow output is displayed rather than the Doppler frequency signal. Power Doppler does not display flow direction or different velocities. It is often used in conjunction with frame averaging to increase sensitivity to low flows and velocities. It complements the other two modes (Table 1). Hybrid color flow modes incorporating power and velocity data are also available from some manufacturers. These can also have improved sensitivity to low flow.

A brief summary of factors influencing the displays in each mode is given in the following sections. Most of these factors are set up approximately for a particular mode

Table 1 Flow imaging modes

Spectral Doppler
Examines flow at one site
Detailed analysis of distribution of flow
Good temporal resolution – can examine flow waveform
Allows calculations of velocity and indices

Color flow
Overall view of flow in a region
Limited flow information
Poor temporal resolution/flow dynamics (frame rate can be low when scanning deep)

Power/energy/amplitude flow
Sensitive to low flows
No directional information in some modes
Very poor temporal resolution
Susceptible to noise

---

when the application (e.g. fetal scan) is chosen, although the operator will usually alter many of the controls during the scan to optimize the image.

Color flow imaging

Color flow Doppler ultrasound produces a color-coded map of Doppler shifts superimposed onto a B-mode ultrasound image (Figure 4b). Although color flow imaging uses pulsed wave ultrasound, its processing differs from that used to provide the Doppler sonogram. Color flow imaging may have to produce several thousand color points of flow information for each frame superimposed on the B-mode image. Color flow imaging uses fewer, shorter pulses along each color scan line of the image to give a mean frequency shift and a variance at each small area of measurement. This frequency shift is displayed as a color pixel. The scanner then repeats this for several lines to build up the color image, which is superimposed onto the B-mode image. The transducer elements are switched rapidly between B-mode and color flow imaging to give an impression of a combined simultaneous image. The pulses used for color flow imaging are typically three to four times longer than those for the B-mode image, with a corresponding loss of axial resolution.

Assignment of color to frequency shifts is usually based on direction (for example, red for Doppler shifts towards the ultrasound beam and blue for shifts away from it) and magnitude (different color hues or lighter saturation for higher frequency shifts). The color Doppler image is dependent on general Doppler factors, particularly the need for a good beam/flow angle. Curvilinear and phased array transducers have a radiating pattern of ultrasound beams that can produce complex color flow images, depending on the orientation of the arteries and veins. In practice, the experienced operator alters the scanning approach to obtain good insonation angles so as to achieve unambiguous flow images.

FACTORS AFFECTING THE COLOR FLOW IMAGE

The controls that affect the appearance of the color flow image are summarized in Table 2. The main factors include:

(1) *Power and gain* Color flow uses higher-intensity power than B-mode. Attention should be paid to safety indices. Power and gain should be set to obtain good signals for flow and to minimize the signals from surrounding tissue.

(2) *Frequency selection* Many scanner/transducer combinations permit changes of frequency. High frequencies give better sensitivity to low flow and have better

Table 2 Factors affecting color flow image

Main factors
Power: transmitted power into tissue*
Gain: overall sensitivity to flow signals
Frequency: trades penetration for sensitivity and resolution*
Pulse repetition frequency (also called scale): low pulse repetition frequency to look at low velocities, high pulse repetition frequency reduces aliasing*
Area of investigation: larger area reduces frame rate*
Focus: color flow image optimized at focal zone*

Other factors
Triplex color: pulse repetition frequency and frame rate reduced by need for B-mode/spectral pulses
Persistence: high persistence produces smoother image but reduces temporal resolution*
Pre-processing: trades resolution against frame rate*
Filter: high filter cuts out more noise but also more of flow signal*
Post-processing assigns color map/variance*

*Settings appropriate for specific examinations assigned by set-up/application keys

spatial resolution. Low frequencies have better penetration (Figure 5) and are less susceptible to aliasing at high velocities.

(3) *Velocity scale/pulse repetition frequency* Low pulse repetition frequencies should be used to examine low velocities but aliasing may occur if high velocities are encountered (Figure 4).

(4) *Region of interest* Because more pulses are needed to look at flow than for the B-mode image, reducing the width and maximum depth of the color flow area under investigation will usually improve frame rate and may allow a higher color scan line density with improved spatial resolution (Figure 6).

(5) *Focus* The focus should be at the level of the area of interest. This can make a significant difference to the appearance and accuracy of the image (Figure 7).

In practice, the operator will make many changes to the controls and will try different probe positions to optimize the image. Practical guidelines are given in Table 3.

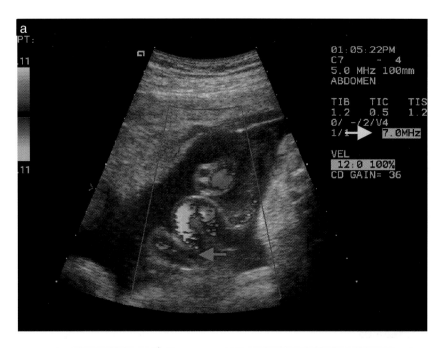

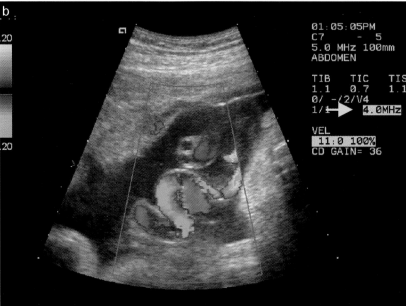

Figure 5 Effect of color flow image transmission frequency. (a) A color flow frequency of 7 MHz is used (yellow arrow). There is poor registration of flow signals in the umbilical cord (red arrow). (b) A lower transmit frequency (4 MHz) is used (yellow arrow). Improved penetration gives better color flow sensitivity

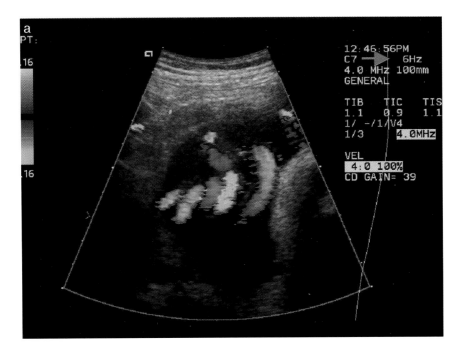

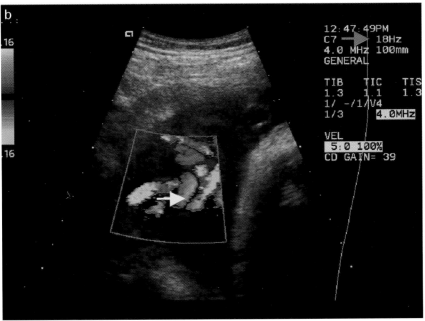

Figure 6 Effect of color flow image region of interest. (a) With a large region of color flow, the frame rate is low (red arrow). The scanner uses a lower density of color flow scan lines. The color images show poor spatial resolution. (b) With a smaller region of interest, the frame rate is improved (red arrow) and there is better definition of the vessels in the color flow image (yellow arrow)

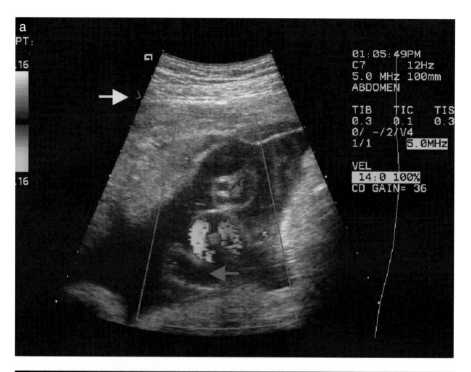

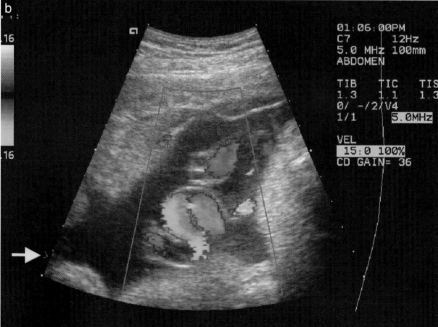

Figure 7 Effect of focus. (a) With the focus set close to the skin (yellow arrow), the color flow image shows poor sensitivity to flow in deeper structures (red arrow). (b) With the focus set deeper (yellow arrow), there is improved color flow sensitivity at depth

Table 3   Color flow imaging: practical guidelines

(1)   Select the appropriate applications/set-up key. This optimizes parameters for specific examinations

(2)   Set power to within fetal study limits. Adjust color gain. Ensure focus is at the region of interest and adjust gain to optimize color signal

(3)   Use probe positioning/beam steering to obtain satisfactory beam/vessel angle

(4)   Adjust pulse repetition frequency/scale to suit the flow conditions. Low pulse repetition frequencies are more sensitive to low flows/velocities but may produce aliasing. High pulse repetition frequencies reduce aliasing but are less sensitive to low velocities

(5)   Set the color flow region to appropriate size. A smaller color flow 'box' may lead to a better frame rate and better color resolution/sensitivity

SPECTRAL OR PULSED WAVE DOPPLER

Pulsed wave Doppler ultrasound is used to provide a sonogram of the artery or vein under investigation (Figure 8). The sonogram provides a measure of the changing velocity throughout the cardiac cycle and the distribution of velocities in the sample volume (or gate) (Figure 9). If an accurate angle correction is made, then absolute velocities can be measured. The best resolution of the sonogram occurs when the B-mode image and color image are frozen, allowing all the time to be employed for spectral Doppler. If concurrent imaging is used (real-time duplex or triplex imaging), the temporal resolution of the sonogram is compromised.

Factors affecting the spectral image

The controls that affect the appearance of the sonogram are summarized in Table 4. The main factors include:

(1)   *Power and gain*   Pulsed wave Doppler uses higher intensity power than B-mode. Attention should be paid to safety indices. Power and gain should be set so that clear signals are obtained.

(2)   *Velocity scale/pulse repetition frequency*   Low pulse repetition frequencies should be used to look at low velocities but aliasing may occur if high velocities are encountered.

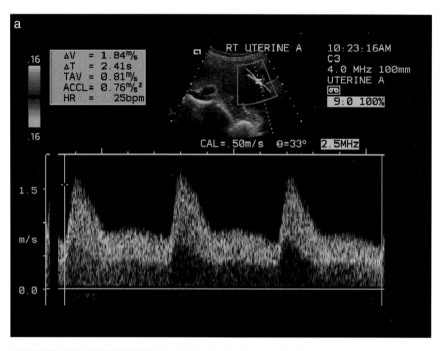

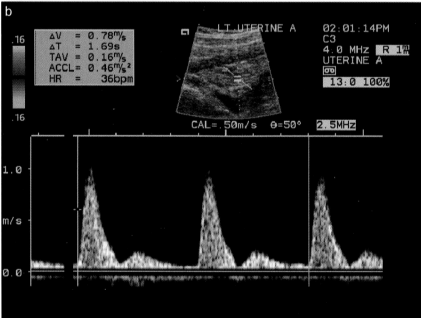

Figure 8 Doppler spectra of uterine artery flow. (a) The color flow image allows beam/flow angle correction. The sonogram shows high velocities throughout the cardiac cycle, indicating low distal resistance. (b) The sonogram shows a pulsatile flow waveform with low diastolic velocities. This is indicative of high distal resistance

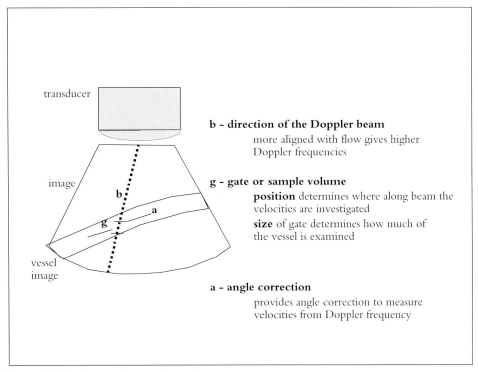

Figure 9 Setting up the sample volume

Table 4 Factors affecting the spectral Doppler image

Main factors

Power: transmitted power into tissue*

Gain: overall sensitivity to flow signals

Pulse repetition frequency (also called scale): low pulse repetition frequency to look at low velocities, high pulse repetition frequency reduces aliasing*

Gate size*

Beam steering can allow improved beam/flow angle for better accuracy of velocity calculation*

Live duplex/triplex spectral resolution constrained by need for B-mode/color pulses

Other factors

Gate: sharpness of resolution*

Filter: high filter cuts out more noise but more of flow signal*

Post-processing: assigns brightness to output*

*Settings appropriate for specific examinations assigned by set-up/application keys

(3) *Gate size*   If flow measurements are being attempted, the whole vessel should be insonated. A large gate may include signals from adjacent vessels (Figure 10).

Guidelines for a practical approach to obtain good-quality spectral images are given in Table 5.

BLOOD FLOW MEASUREMENTS

Velocity measurement

Theoretically, once the beam/flow angle is known, velocities can be calculated from the Doppler spectrum as shown in the Doppler equation. However, errors in the measured velocity may still occur[1,4]. Sources of error can be broadly divided into three categories.

(1) Errors can arise in the formation of the Doppler spectrum due to:

    (a) Use of multiple elements in array transducers;
    (b) Non-uniform insonation of the vessel lumen;
    (c) Insonation of more than one vessel;
    (d) Use of filters removing low-velocity components.

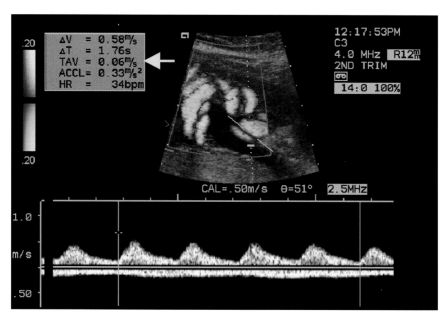

Figure 10   Influence of gate size. The spectral Doppler gate insonates an artery and vein and the sonogram shows flow from both of these vessels. The calculation of mean velocity (arrow) is meaningless since velocities from one vessel subtract from those of the other

18

Table 5   Spectral Doppler imaging: practical guidelines

(1)   Set power to within fetal study limits

(2)   Position the pulsed wave Doppler cursor on the vessel to be investigated

(3)   Adjust gain so that the sonogram is clearly visible and free of noise

(4)   Use probe positioning/beam steering to obtain a satisfactory beam/vessel angle. Angles close to 90° will give ambiguous/unclear values. The beam/vessel angle should be 60° or less if velocity measurements are to be made

(5)   Adjust the pulse repetition frequency/scale and baseline to suit flow conditions. The sonogram should be clear and not aliased

(6)   Set the sample volume to correct size. Correct the angle to obtain accurate velocities. Use the B-mode and color flow image of the vessel to make the angle correction

(2)   Errors can arise in the measurement of the ultrasound beam/flow velocity angle. Use of high angles ($\theta > 60°$) may give rise to error because of the comparatively large changes in the cosine of the angle which occur with small changes of angle (Figure 11). The velocity vector may not be in the direction of the vessel axis.

(3)   Errors can arise in the calculation packages provided by the manufacturers for analysis of the Doppler spectrum (for instance, of intensity weighted mean velocity). While efforts can be made to minimize errors, the operator should be aware of their likely range. It is good practice to try to repeat velocity measurements, if possible using a different beam approach, to gain a feel for the variability of measurements in a particular application. However, even repeated measurements may not reveal systematic errors occurring in a particular machine.

The effort applied to produce accurate velocity measurements should be balanced against the importance of absolute velocity measurements for an investigation. Changes in velocity and velocity waveform shape are often of more clinical relevance when making a diagnosis. In this and other cases, absolute values of velocity measurement may not be required.

Calculation of absolute flow

Total flow measurement using color or duplex Doppler ultrasound is fraught with difficulties, even under ideal conditions[5]. Errors that may arise include:

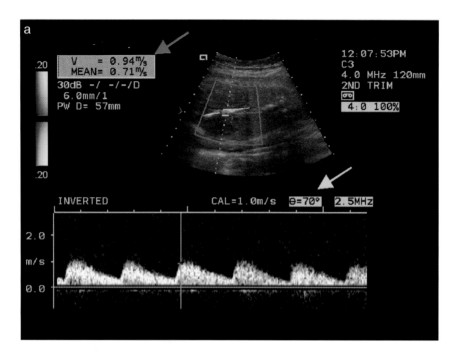

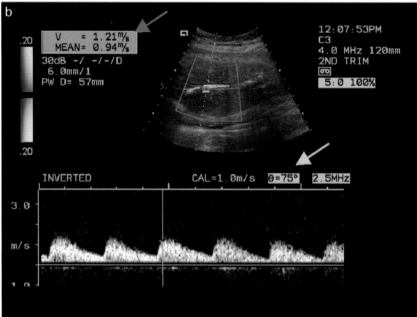

Figure 11   Effect of high vessel/beam angles. (a) and (b) A scan of fetal aortic flow is undertaken at a high beam/vessel angle. Both beam/vessel angle corrections are plausible but a 5° difference in angle (yellow arrows) yields a measured velocity discrepancy of over 25% (red arrows). If absolute velocities are to be measured, beam/flow angles should be kept to 60° or less

(1) Those due to inaccurate measurement of vessel cross-sectional area, for example the cross-sectional area of arteries which pulsate during the cardiac cycle;

(2) Those originating in the derivation of velocity (see above).

These errors become particularly large when flow calculations are made in small vessels; errors in measurement of diameter are magnified when the diameter is used to derive cross-sectional area. As with velocity measurements, it is prudent to be aware of possible errors and to conduct repeatability tests.

Flow waveform analysis

Non-dimensional analysis of the flow waveform shape and spectrum has proved to be a useful technique in the investigation of many vascular beds. It has the advantage that derived indices are independent of the beam/flow angle.

Changes in flow waveform shape have been used to investigate both proximal disease (e.g. in the adult peripheral arterial circulation) and distal changes (in the fetal circulation and uterine arteries). While the breadth of possible uses shows the technique to be versatile, it also serves as a reminder of the range of factors which cause changes to the local Doppler spectrum. If waveform analysis is to be used to observe changes in one component of the proximal or distal vasculature, consideration must be given to what effects other components may have on the waveform.

Flow waveform shape: indices of measurement

Many different indices have been used to describe the shape of flow waveforms[1]. Techniques range from simple indices of systolic to diastolic flow to feature extraction methods such as principal component analysis. All are designed to describe the waveform in a quantitative way, usually as a guide to some kind of classification. In general, they are a compromise between simplicity and the amount of information obtained. The relative merits of indices used in uterine arteries have been discussed elsewhere[6,7].

Commonly used indices available on most commercial scanners are:

(1) Resistance index (RI) (also called resistive index or Pourcelot's index);

(2) Systolic/diastolic (S/D) ratio, sometimes called the A/B ratio;

(3) Pulsatility index (PI)[8].

These indices are all based on the maximum Doppler shift waveform and their calculation is described in Figure 12. The PI takes slightly longer to calculate than the RI or S/D ratio because of the need to measure the mean height of the waveform. It does, however, give a broader range of values, for instance in describing a range of waveform shapes when there is no end-diastolic flow.

In addition to these indices, the flow waveform may be described or categorized by the presence or absence of a particular feature, for example the absence of end-diastolic flow and the presence of a post-systolic notch.

Generally, a low pulsatility waveform is indicative of low distal resistance and high pulsatility waveforms occur in high-resistance vascular beds (Figure 8), although the presence of proximal stenosis, vascular steal or arteriovenous fistulas can modify waveform shape. Care should be taken when trying to interpret indices as absolute measurements of either upstream or downstream factors. For example, alterations in heart rate can alter the flow waveform shape and cause significant changes in the value of indices.

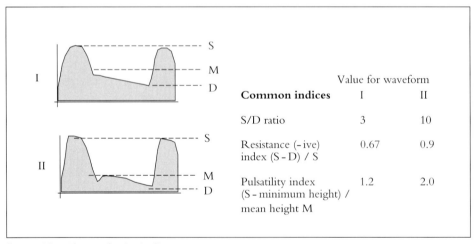

Common indices	Value for waveform I	II
S/D ratio	3	10
Resistance (-ive) index (S - D) / S	0.67	0.9
Pulsatility index (S - minimum height) / mean height M	1.2	2.0

Figure 12   Flow velocity indices

REFERENCES

1. Evans DH, McDicken WN, Skidmore R, Woodcock JP. *Doppler Ultrasound: Physics, Instrumentation, and Clinical Applications*. Chichester: Wiley, 1989
2. Powis RL, Schwartz RD. *Practical Doppler Ultrasound for the Clinician*. Williams and Wilkins, 1991
3. Goldberg BB, Merton DA, Deane CR. *An Atlas of Ultrasound Color Flow Imaging*. London: Martin Dunitz, 1997

4. Gill RW. Measurement of blood flow by ultrasound: accuracy and sources of error. *Ultrasound Med Biol* 1985;7:625–42

5. Rourke C, Hendrickx P, Roth U, Brassel F, Creutzig A, Alexander K. Color and conventional image-directed ultrasonography: accuracy and sources of error in quantitative blood flow measurement. *J Clin Ultrasound* 1992;20:187–93

6. Thompson RS, Trudinger BJ, Cook CM. A comparison of Doppler ultrasound waveform indices in the umbilical artery. I. Indices derived from the maximum velocity waveform. *Ultrasound Med Biol* 1986;12:835–44

7. Thompson RS, Trudinger BJ, Cook CM. A comparison of Doppler ultrasound waveform indices in the umbilical artery. II. Indices derived from the mean velocity and first moment waveforms. *Ultrasound Med Biol* 1986;12:845–54

8. Gosling RG, King DH. Continuous wave ultrasound as an alternative and complement to X-rays in vascular examination. In Reneman RS, ed. *Cardiovascular Applications of Ultrasound*. Amsterdam: North Holland, 1974:266–82

2

Safety of diagnostic ultrasound in fetal scanning

Colin Deane

INTRODUCTION

Diagnostic ultrasound is generally perceived by users and patients as a safe technique with no adverse effects. Since ultrasound is so widely used in pregnancy, it is essential for all practitioners to ensure that its use remains safe. Ultrasound causes thermal and mechanical effects in tissue which are increased as the output power is increased.

In the last decade, there has been a general trend towards increased output with the introduction of color flow imaging, more use of pulsed 'spectral Doppler' and higher demands on B-mode imaging[1]. In response to these increases, recommendations for the safe use of ultrasound have been issued by several bodies. In addition, recent regulations have changed the emphasis of responsibility so that more onus is now placed on the operator to ensure that ultrasound is used safely. This chapter summarizes the effects and the standards issued and outlines recommendations for safe use in obstetric practice.

EFFECTS

Ultrasound is a mechanical energy in which a pressure wave travels through tissue. Reflection and scattering back to the transducer are used to form the image. The physical effects of ultrasound are generally categorized as:

(1) Thermal effects – heating of tissue as ultrasound is absorbed by tissue. Heat is also produced at the transducer surface;

(2) Cavitation – the formation of gas bubbles at high negative pressure;

(3) Other mechanical effects – radiation forces leading to streaming in fluids and stress at tissue interfaces.

The implications of these effects have been determined by *in vitro*, animal and human epidemiological studies and are briefly summarized below.

Thermal effects

As the ultrasound waves are absorbed, their energy is converted into heat. The level of conversion is highest in tissue with a high absorption coefficient, particularly in bone, and is low where there is little absorption (e.g. amniotic fluid). The temperature rise is also dependent on the thermal characteristics of the tissue (conduction of heat and perfusion), the ultrasound intensity and the length of time for which the tissue volume is scanned. The intensity is, in turn, dependent on the power output and the position of the tissue in the beam profile. The intensity at a particular point is altered by many of the operator controls, for example power output, mode (B-mode, color flow, spectral Doppler), scan depth, focus, zoom and area of color flow imaging.

With so many variables, it has proved difficult to model temperature rises in tissue. *In vitro* studies have been used with a 'worst case' model of tissue to predict temperature rises *in vivo*, for instance in the formation of thermal indices (see below).

The *transducer face* itself can become heated during an examination. Heat is localized to the tissue in contact with the transducer.

Cavitation

Cavitation is the formation of transient or stable bubbles, described as inertial or non-inertial cavitation. Inertial cavitation has the most potential to damage tissue and occurs when a gas-filled cavity grows, during pressure rarefaction of the ultrasound pulse, and contracts, during the compression phase. Collapse of the bubble can generate local high temperatures and pressures.

It has been hypothesized that ultrasonically induced cavitation is the cause of hemorrhage in the lungs and intestines in animal studies[2-6]. In these studies, effects have been seen at tissue interfaces with gas. The absence of gas in fetuses means that the threshold for cavitation is high and does not occur at current levels of diagnostic ultrasound. The introduction of contrast agents leads to the formation of microbubbles that potentially provide gas nuclei for cavitation. The use of contrast agents lowers the threshold at which cavitation occurs, but this is not current practice in obstetrics.

Other mechanical effects

The passage of ultrasound through tissue causes a low-level radiation force on the tissue. This force produces a pressure in the direction of the beam and away from the transducer and should not be confused with the oscillatory pressure of the ultrasound itself. The pressure that results and the pressure gradient across the beam are very low, even for intensities at the higher end of the diagnostic range[7].

The effect of the force is manifest in volumes of fluid where *streaming* can occur with motion within the fluid. The fluid velocities which result are low and are unlikely to cause damage.

Effects on fetuses

Effects are divided into mechanical and thermal. For mechanical effects, there is no evidence that cavitation occurs in fetal scanning. In a study of low-amplitude lithotripsy pulses in mouse fetuses, there has been concern that hemorrhage may be the result of tissue movement caused by radiation forces[8]. There is no evidence that this occurs *in vivo* in fetal scanning.

The primary concern in fetal imaging is temperature rise. It is known that hyperthermia is teratogenic. The efforts of investigators have concentrated on defining the temperature increases and exposure times which may give rise to biological effects and on determining the ultrasound levels which might, in turn, lead to those temperature rises. With this information, criteria have been identified for the safe use of diagnostic ultrasound.

Temperature rises of 2.5°C have been demonstrated in excised unperfused guinea pig brain tissue after 2 minutes' exposure to ultrasound at the high end of pulsed wave Doppler ultrasound intensity levels[9]. At the bone surface, temperature increases of up to 5°C were found. In a study on sheep using different intensity criteria[10], the temperature rise *in utero* was found to be 40% lower than that in the equivalent non-perfused test. While the observed temperature increases occurred in high-intensity modes (typical of pulsed wave Doppler used at maximum power), these levels of intensity are achievable with some current scanner/transducer combinations.

The issue of sensitivity of fetal tissue to temperature rise is complex and is not completely understood. Acute and chronic temperature rises have been investigated in animals, but study designs and results are varied. Work carried out in this field is summarized elsewhere[11].

The uncertainty over chronic changes is reflected in the WFUMB guidelines[12]. These state that ultrasound that produces temperature rises of less than 1.5°C may be used without reservation. They also state that ultrasound exposure causing temperature rises of greater than 4°C for over 5 min should be considered potentially hazardous. This leaves a wide range of temperature increases which are within the capability of diagnostic ultrasound equipment to produce and for which no time limits are recommended.

Epidemiology

Several studies have examined the development of fetuses receiving different levels of ultrasound investigation. In trials comparing ultrasound screened and non-screened groups, there has generally been no difference in birth weights between groups. There have been no unequivocal data to suggest that there is impaired development of hearing, vision, behavior or neurological function due to ultrasound screening.

In a large, randomized trial of over 3200 pregnant women in which half were offered routine ultrasonography at 19 and 32 weeks, there was no evidence of impaired growth or neurological development up to follow-up at 8–9 years. There was a possible association of left-handedness amongst boys undergoing ultrasonography[13]. Scanning of this group was performed with B-mode only. There have been concerns that epidemiological studies to date do not reflect the higher output capabilities of modern scanners.

OUTPUT REGULATIONS, STANDARDS AND GUIDELINES – WHO DOES WHAT?

Regulations governing the output of diagnostic ultrasound have been largely set by the USA's Food and Drug Administration (FDA), although the International Electrotechnical Commission (IEC) is currently in the process of setting internationally agreed standards.

The relevant national societies for ultrasound users (e.g. American Institutue of Ultrasound in Medicine (AIUM), British Medical Ultrasound Society (BMUS)) usually have safety committees who offer *advice* on the safe use of ultrasound. In 1992, the AIUM, in conjunction with the National Electrical Manufacturers Association (NEMA) developed the Output Display Standard (ODS), including the thermal index and mechanical index which have been incorporated in the FDA's new regulations[14,15].

Within Europe, the Federation of Societies of Ultrasound in Medicine and Biology (EFSUMB) also addresses safety and has produced safety guidelines (through the European Committee for Ultrasound Radiation Safety). The World Federation (WFUMB) held safety symposia in 1991 (on thermal issues) and 1996 (thermal and non-thermal issues), at which recommendations were proffered. Following review, these were published in 1992 and 1998 as guidelines.

Past regulations

The initial FDA regulations on ultrasound output were produced in 1976. These imposed application-specific limits, based on existing output levels which had demonstrated no adverse effects. Limits were divided into:

(1) Ophthalmic applications;

(2) Fetal and other (including abdominal, pediatric, small parts);

(3) Cardiac;

(4) Peripheral vessels.

For spatial peak time-averaged intensity (I-SPTA) (the measure most associated with temperature rise), the maximum levels were:

Ophthalmic	17 mW/cm^2
Fetal and other	94 mW/cm^2
Cardiac	430 mW/cm^2
Peripheral vessel	720 mW/cm^2

Scanners typically had a key/button which limited output for obstetric applications. Although power and intensity limits could be exceeded in some scanners, especially when using pulsed wave Doppler or color Doppler, this required a deliberate effort on the behalf of the users.

Current regulations

In revising its regulations in 1993, the FDA[15] altered its approach to ultrasound safety. The new regulations combine an overall limit of I-SPTA of 720 mW/cm² for all equipment with a system of output displays to allow users to employ effective and judicious levels of ultrasound appropriate to the examination undertaken.

The new regulations allow an eight-fold increase in ultrasound intensity to be used in fetal examinations. They place considerably more responsibility on the user to understand the output measurements and to use them in their scanning.

The output display is based on two indices, the mechanical index (MI) and the thermal index (TI).

Mechanical index

The mechanical index is an estimate of the maximum amplitude of the pressure pulse in tissue. It gives an indication as to the relative risk of mechanical effects (streaming and cavitation). The FDA regulations allow a mechanical index of up to 1.9 to be used for all applications except ophthalmic (maximum 0.23).

Thermal index

The thermal index is the ratio of the power used to that required to cause a maximum temperature increase of 1°C. A thermal index of 1 indicates a power causing a temperature increase of 1°C. A thermal index of 2 would be twice that power but would not necessarily indicate a peak temperature rise of 2°C. Because temperature rise is dependent on tissue type and is particularly dependent on the presence of bone, the thermal index is subdivided into three indices:

(1) TIS: thermal index for soft tissue;

(2) TIB: thermal index with bone at/near the focus;

(3) TIC: thermal index with bone at the surface (e.g. cranial examination).

For fetal scanning, the highest temperature increase would be expected to occur at bone and TIB would give the 'worst case' conditions. The mechanical index and thermal index must be displayed if the ultrasound system is capable of exceeding an index of 1. The displayed indices are based on the manufacturer's experimental and modelled data. These measurements are not infallible; an independent study has demonstrated significant discrepancies over declared I-SPTA output of up to 400%[16].

Future IEC standards

An IEC standard (Draft IEC 61681) is being drawn up to establish a safety classification for ultrasound equipment based on its ability to produce cavitation or a temperature rise. The standard proposes two classifications of equipment: class A, which has a lower output and for which no output display is required, and class B which has a higher output and for which an output display is required. The draft is currently undergoing review.

Guidelines

Ultrasound organizations have produced statements on the safe use of ultrasound. These are not regulatory statements but are intended to educate and advise.

WFUMB guidelines have been issued in two special issues of *Ultrasound in Medicine and Biology*[12,17]. Statements and recommendations are given on B-mode scanning, Doppler imaging, transducer heating, thermal effects (see page 33). The AIUM have produced statements on the safety of ultrasound. They are available from the AIUM office and can be obtained from the AIUM website – http://www.aium.org/stmts.htm.

The European Committee for Ultrasound Radiation Safety has published statements[18,19] on the use of pulsed Doppler measurement in fetuses, stating that its use in routine examinations during the period of organogenesis is considered inadvisable at present.

A PRACTICAL APPROACH TO SAFE FETAL SCANNING

No injurious effects have been identified from ultrasound scanning of the fetus. However, changes in power output, increased use of Doppler ultrasound and a change in regulations governing outputs means that every measure should be taken by users to maintain safe practices.

Scanning practice

● The ALARA (as low as reasonably achievable) principle should be maintained. Power outputs used should be adequate to conduct the examination. If in doubt, use a low power and increase it as necessary. Application keys for obstetrics should bring in each mode at its lowest output so that the operator is required to increase power if the examination demands it.

- B-mode generally has the lowest power output and intensity. M-mode, color flow and spectral Doppler have higher outputs which can cause more heating at the site of examination. The examination should begin with B-mode and use color and spectral Doppler only when necessary.

- The intensity (and temperature rise) is highly dependent on scanner settings. For example, the intensity changes in response to changes in:

  (a) Power output,

  (b) Depth of examination,

  (c) Mode used (color flow, spectral Doppler),

  (d) Transmitted frequency used,

  (e) Color pulse repetition frequency (scale),

  (f) Region of color flow interest,

  (g) Focus.

  If the display for the scanner/transducer combination shows thermal and mechanical indices, the indices should be readily visible. Of the thermal indices, TIB is most relevant to heating in the second and third trimesters. The operator should be aware of changes to the indices in response to changes in control settings.

- Special care should be taken in febrile patients, since ultrasound heating will cause additional heating to the fetus.

- The WFUMB recommends that ultrasound causing a temperature rise of no more than 1.5°C may be used without reservation on thermal grounds.

- Thermal indices exceeding 1.5 should not be used routinely and, if required for specific diagnostic information, should be used for the minimum time necessary. The influence of higher intensity levels can be moderated by moving the transducer so that specific areas of tissue are not subjected to long periods of higher intensity investigation.

- Do not scan for longer than is necessary to obtain the diagnostic information.

SELECTED WFUMB STATEMENTS ON THE SAFETY OF DIAGNOSTIC ULTRASOUND

B-mode imaging (issued 1992)

Known diagnostic ultrasound equipment as used today for simple B-mode imaging operates at acoustic outputs that are not capable of producing harmful temperature rises. Its use in medicine is therefore not contraindicated on thermal grounds. This includes endoscopic, transvaginal and transcutaneous applications.

Doppler (1992)

It has been demonstrated in experiments with unperfused tissue that some Doppler diagnostic equipment has the potential to produce biologically significant temperature rises, specifically at bone/soft tissue interfaces. The effects of elevated temperatures may be minimized by keeping the time during which the beam passes through any one point in tissue as short as possible. Where output power can be controlled, the lowest available power level consistent with obtaining the desired diagnostic information should be used.

Although the data on humans are sparse, it is clear from animal studies that exposures resulting in temperatures less than 38.5°C can be used without reservation on thermal grounds. This includes obstetric applications.

Transducer heating (1992)

A substantial source of heating may be the transducer itself. Tissue heating from this source is localized to the volume in contact with the transducer.

Recommendations on thermal effects (1997)

A diagnostic exposure that produces a maximum temperature rise of no more than 1.5°C above normal physiological levels (37°C) may be used without reservation on thermal grounds.

A diagnostic exposure that elevates embryonic and fetal *in situ* temperature to 41°C (4°C above normal temperature) for 5 min or more should be considered potentially hazardous.

REFERENCES

1. Henderson J, Willson K, Jago JR, *et al.* A survey of the acoustic outputs of diagnostic ultrasound equipment in current clinical use in the Northern Region. *Ultrasound Med Biol* 1995;21:699–705

2. Baggs R, Penney DP, Cox C, Child SZ. Thresholds for ultrasonically induced lung hemorrhage in neonatal swine. *Ultrasound Med Biol* 1996;22:119–28

3. Dalecki D, Child SZ, Raeman CH, Cox C, Carstensen EL. Ultrasonically-induced lung haemorrhage in young swine. *Ultrasound Med Biol* 1997;23:777–81

4. Frizzell LA, Chen E, Chong L. Effects of pulsed ultrasound on the mouse neonate: hind limb paralysis and lung haemorrhage. *Ultrasound Med Biol* 1994;20:53–63

5. Holland CK, Zheng X, Apfel RE, Alderman JL, Fernandez L, Taylor KJW. Direct evidence of cavitation *in vivo* from diagnostic ultrasound. *Ultrasound Med Biol* 1996;22:917–25

6. Zacchary JG, O'Brien WD. Lung lesions induced by continuous and pulsed wave (diagnostic) ultrasound in mice, rabbits and pigs. *Vet Pathol* 1995;32:43–54

7. Duck FA. Acoustic streaming and radiation pressure in diagnostic applications: what are the implications? In Barnett SB, Kossoff G, eds. *Safety of Diagnostic Ultrasound*. Carnforth, UK: Parthenon Publishing, 1998:87–98

8. Dalecki D, Child SZ, Raeman CH, Penney DP, Mayer R, Cox C, Carstensen EL. Thresholds for fetal haemorrhages produced by a piezoelectric lithotripter. *Ultrasound Med Biol* 1997;23:287–97

9. Bosward KL, Barnett SB, Wood AKW, Edwards MJ, Kossoff G. Heating of the guinea pig fetal brain during exposure to pulsed ultrasound. *Ultrasound Med Biol* 1993;19:415–24

10. Duggan PM, Liggins GC, Barnett SB. Ultrasonic heating of the brain of the fetal sheep in utero. *Ultrasound Med Biol* 1995;21:553–60

11. Tarantal AF. Effects of ultrasound exposure on fetal development in animal models. In Barnett SB, Kossoff G, eds. *Safety of Diagnostic Ultrasound*. Carnforth, UK: Parthenon Publishing, 1998:39–51

12. Barnett SB, ed. Conclusions and recommendations on thermal and non-thermal mechanisms for biological effects of ultrasound. In *WFUMB symposium on Safety of Ultrasound in Medicine*. *Ultrasound Med Biol*, 1998;24, special issue

13. Salveson K, Vatten L, Eik-Nes S, Hugdahl K, Bakketeig L. Routine ultrasonography *in utero* and subsequent handedness and neurological development. *Br Med J* 1993;307:159–64

14. AIUM / NEMA. *Standard for Real-Time Display of Thermal and Mechanical Acoustic Output Indices on Diagnostic Ultrasound Equipment*. Rockville: American Institute of Ultrasound in Medicine, 1992

15. FDA. *Revised 510(k) Diagnostic Ultrasound Guidance for 1993*. Rockville, MD: Food and Drug Administration, Center for Devices and Radiological Health, 1993

16. Jago JR, Henderson J, Whittingham TA, Willson K. How reliable are manufacturer's reported acoustic output data? *Ultrasound Med Biol* 1995;12:135–6

17. Barnett SB, Kossoff G. eds. Issues and recommendations regarding thermal mechanisms for biological effects of ultrasound. In *WFUMB Symposium on Safety and Standardization in Medical Ultrasound*. *Ultrasound Med Biol* 1992;18, special issue

18. European Federation of Societies for Ultrasound in Medicine and Biology. *Guidelines for the safe use of Doppler ultrasound for clinical applications*. Report from the European Committee for Ultrasound Radiation Safety. *Eur J Ultrasound* 1995;2:167–8

19. European Federation of Societies for Ultrasound in Medicine and Biology. *Clinical safety statement for diagnostic ultrasound*. Report from the European Committee for Ultrasound Radiation Safety. *Eur J Ultrasound* 1996;3:283

3

Methodology of Doppler assessment of the placental and fetal circulations

Doppler ultrasound provides a non-invasive method for the study of fetal hemodynamics. Investigation of the uterine and umbilical arteries gives information on the perfusion of the uteroplacental and fetoplacental circulations, respectively, while Doppler studies of selected fetal organs are valuable in detecting the hemodynamic re-arrangements that occur in response to fetal hypoxemia.

FACTORS AFFECTING FLOW VELOCITY WAVEFORM

Maternal position

During Doppler studies, the mother should lie in a semirecumbent position with a slight lateral tilt. This minimizes the risk of developing supine hypotension syndrome due to caval compression.

Fetal heart rate

There is an inverse relation between fetal heart rate and length of cardiac cycle and, therefore, fetal heart rate influences the configuration of the arterial Doppler waveform. When the heart rate drops, the diastolic phase of the cardiac cycle is prolonged and the end-diastolic frequency shift declines. Although the Doppler indices are affected by the fetal heart rate, the change is of no clinical significance when the rate is within the normal range.

Fetal breathing movements

During fetal breathing movements, there are variations in the shape of the flow velocity waveforms from fetal vessels and, therefore, Doppler examinations should be conducted only during fetal apnea and in the absence of fetal hiccup or excessive movement.

Blood viscosity

Animal studies have demonstrated that increased blood viscosity is associated with reduced cardiac output and increased peripheral resistance, and vice versa. However, Giles *et al.* were unable to demonstrate a significant association between blood viscosity (measured in post-delivery umbilical cord blood) and impedance to flow in the umbilical artery[1].

UTEROPLACENTAL CIRCULATION

Anatomy

The blood supply to the uterus comes mainly from the uterine arteries, with a small contribution from the ovarian arteries. These vessels anastomose at the cornu of the uterus and give rise to arcuate arteries that run circumferentially round the uterus. The radial arteries arise from the arcuate vessels and penetrate at right angles into the outer third of the myometrium. These vessels then give rise to the basal and spiral arteries, which nourish the myometrium and decidua and the intervillous space of the placenta during pregnancy, respectively. There are about 100 functional openings of spiral arteries into the intervillous space in a mature placenta, but maternal blood enters the space in discrete spurts from only a few of these[2,3].

Physiological changes in pregnancy

Physiological modification of spiral arteries is required to permit the ten-fold increase in uterine blood flow which is necessary to meet the respiratory and nutritional requirements of the fetus and placenta. Brosens *et al.* examined microscopically several hundred placental bed biopsies, seven Cesarean hysterectomy specimens and two intact second-trimester uteri[4]. Basal arteries showed no changes, but spiral arteries were invaded by cytotrophoblastic cells and were converted into uteroplacental arteries. These have a dilated and tortuous lumen, a complete absence of muscular and elastic tissue, no continuous endothelial lining, mural thrombi and fibrinoid deposition.

This conversion of the spiral arteries to uteroplacental arteries is termed 'physiological change'. It has been reported to occur in two stages: the first wave of trophoblastic invasion converts the decidual segments of the spiral arteries in the first trimester and the second wave converts the myometrial segments in the second trimester[5]. As a result of this 'physiological change', the diameter of the spiral arteries increases from 15–20 to 300–500 μm, thus reducing impedance to flow and optimizing fetomaternal exchange in the intervillous space.

Invasive assessment of blood flow

Assali *et al.* measured uterine blood flow by placing electromagnetic flow meters in the uterine vessels at the time of hysterotomy for termination of pregnancy and demonstrated that both uterine blood flow and oxygen consumption increase with gestation[6]. Browne and Veall injected [24]Na tracer directly into the choriodecidual space of women with anterior placentae and used a Geiger counter to construct decay curves for the falling levels of radioactivity[7]. Although this method was beset by technical failures, it established the commonly quoted figure of 600 ml/min for uterine blood flow at term.

Methodology of obtaining waveforms

Campbell *et al.* used pulsed wave Doppler to obtain velocity waveforms from 'arcuate' arteries, which were described as vessels in the wall of the uterus distinct from the common, internal and external iliac arteries[8]. Trudinger *et al.* described the use of continuous wave Doppler to obtain velocity waveforms from branches of the uterine artery in the placental bed[9]. The placental site was located using real-time ultrasound and the Doppler probe was then pointed at the center of the placental bed and 'searched' until characteristic waveforms were obtained. Validation of the method was performed by directing a pulsed wave Doppler facility along the same line and obtaining identical waveforms from subplacental vessels.

Schulman *et al.* described the use of continuous wave Doppler ultrasound to locate the uterine artery[10]. The Doppler probe was directed into the parauterine area in the region of the lower uterine segment and rotated until a characteristic waveform pattern was recognized. In the early stages of the study, the methodology was validated with Duplex equipment or by *in vivo* measurements obtained during Cesarean section. They found that patterns of uterine, arcuate and iliac vessels could be differentiated from each other and from other vessels in the pelvis. The presence of an early diastolic notch was noted and was found to disappear between 20 and 26 weeks.

Bewley *et al.* used continuous wave Doppler to obtain flow velocity waveforms from four fixed points on the uterus[11]. The two lower 'uterine' sites were insonated in a similar way to that described by Schulman *et al.*[10], except that the transducer was pointed medially and caudally about 2 cm above and halfway along the inguinal ligament on either side of the uterus. The two upper 'arcuate' sites were halfway between the fundus of the uterus and its most lateral point.

Arduini *et al.* compared color flow imaging and conventional pulsed Doppler in the study of the uterine artery[12]. Color flow imaging was used to visualize the flow through the main uterine artery medial to the external iliac artery (Figure 1) and the Doppler sample gate was placed at the point of maximal color brightness. Color flow imaging was found to allow a higher number of reliable recordings to be obtained, to shorten the observation time, and to reduce the intra- and interobserver coefficients of variation.

Impedance to flow in the uterine arteries decreases with gestation (Figure 2). The initial fall until 24–26 weeks is thought to be due to trophoblastic invasion of the spiral arteries, but a continuing fall in impedance may be explained in part by a persisting hormonal effect on elasticity of arterial walls. Impedance in the uterine artery on the same site as the placenta is lower, which is thought to be due to the trophoblastic invasion only taking place in placental spiral arteries and the fall in impedance engendered by this being transmitted to other parts of the uterine circulation through collaterals. The intra- and interobserver coefficients of variation in the measurement of impedance to flow from the uterine arteries are both 5–10%.

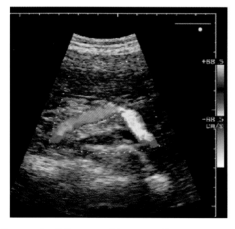 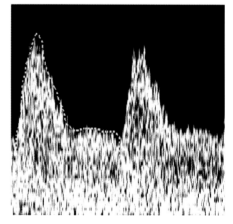

Figure 1 Ultrasound image with superimposed color Doppler showing the uterine artery and the external iliac artery (left). Normal flow velocity waveforms from the uterine artery at 24 weeks of gestation demonstrating high diastolic flow (right)

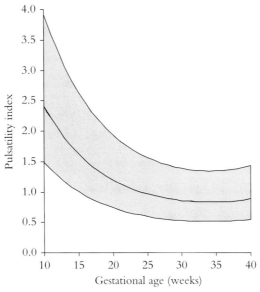

Figure 2 Pulsatility index in the uterine artery with gestation (mean 95th and 5th centiles)

UMBILICAL ARTERY FLOW

The umbilical artery was the first fetal vessel to be evaluated by Doppler velocimetry. Flow velocity waveforms from the umbilical cord have a characteristic saw-tooth appearance of arterial flow in one direction and continuous umbilical venous blood flow in the other. Continuous wave Doppler examination of the umbilical artery is simple. The transducer, usually a pencil-shaped probe, is placed on the mother's abdomen overlying the fetus and is systematically manipulated to obtain the characteristic waveforms from the umbilical artery and vein. With a pulsed wave Doppler system, an ultrasound scan is first carried out, a free-floating portion of the cord is identified and the Doppler sample volume is placed over an artery and the vein (Figure 3).

The location of the Doppler sampling site in the umbilical cord affects the Doppler waveform and the impedance indices are significantly higher at the fetal end of the cord than at the placental end. A possible explanation for this finding is that the fetal placental vascular bed is a low impedance system associated with minimal wave reflection, which explains the presence of continuing forward flow in the umbilical artery during diastole. The closer the measurement site is to the placenta, the less is the wave reflection and the greater the end-diastolic flow. Consequently, the Doppler waveform that represents arterial flow velocity demonstrates progressively declining pulsatility and the indices of pulsatility from the fetal to the placental end of the cord[13].

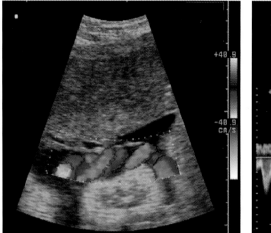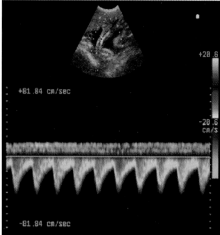

Figure 3 Ultrasound image with superimposed color Doppler showing the umbilical cord (left). Normal flow velocity waveforms from the umbilical vein (top) and artery (bottom) at 32 weeks of gestation (right)

There are no appreciable diurnal changes or significant day-to-day variations in pregnancies with normal umbilical arterial Doppler waveforms. Umbilical venous blood flow increases with fetal inspiration (during which the fetal abdominal wall moves inward) and decreases with expiration (during which the wall moves outward). There is also a breathing-related modulation of arterial pulsatility, and umbilical artery Doppler studies should be avoided during fetal breathing. Maternal exercise may cause an increase in fetal heart rate but mild to moderate exercise does not affect flow impedance in the umbilical artery. Umbilical arterial flow waveforms are not affected by fetal behavioral states (sleep or wakefulness). Although, in certain pregnancy disorders (such as pre-eclampsia), fetal blood viscosity is increased, the contribution to the increased impedance in the umbilical artery from viscosity is minimal compared to the coexisting placental pathology. Therefore, the viscosity of fetal blood need not be considered when interpreting the umbilical Doppler indices.

With advancing gestation, umbilical arterial Doppler waveforms demonstrate a progressive rise in the end-diastolic velocity and a decrease in the impedance indices (Figure 4). When the high-pass filter is either turned off or set at the lowest value, end-diastolic frequencies may be detected from as early as 10 weeks and in normal pregnancies they are always present from 15 weeks. Human placental studies have demonstrated that there is continuing expansion of the fetoplacental vascular system throughout the pregnancy. Furthermore, the villous vascular system undergoes a transformation, resulting in the appearance of sinusoidal dilatation in the terminal villous

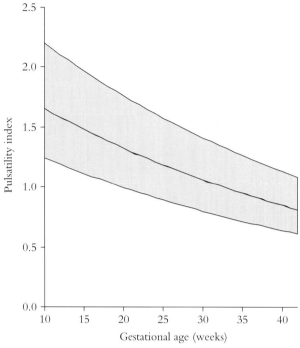

Figure 4 Pulsatility index in the umbilical artery with gestation (mean, 95th and 5th centiles)

capillaries as pregnancy approaches term, and more than 50% of the stromal volume may be vascularized. The intra- and interobserver variations in the various indices are about 5% and 10%, respectively[14].

FETAL ARTERIAL FLOW

Descending aorta

Velocity waveforms from the fetal descending aorta are usually recorded at the lower thoracic level just above the diaphragm, keeping the angle of insonation of the Doppler beam below 45° (Figure 5). It may be difficult to obtain a low angle because the aorta runs anterior to the fetal spine and, therefore, parallel to the surface of the maternal abdomen. This problem can be overcome, by moving the transducer either toward the fetal head or toward its breech and then tilting the transducer.

Diastolic velocities are always present during the second and third trimesters of normal pregnancy, and the pulsatility index (PI) remains constant throughout gestation (Figure 6)[15]. Flow velocity waveforms in the descending aorta represent the summation

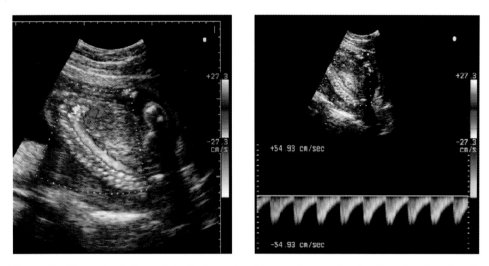

Figure 5 Parasagittal view of the fetal trunk with superimposed color Doppler showing the descending aorta (left). Flow velocity waveforms from the fetal descending aorta at 32 weeks of gestation demonstrating positive end-diastolic velocities (right)

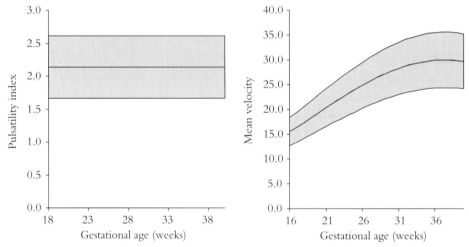

Figure 6 Pulsatility index (left) and mean blood velocity (right) in the fetal aorta with gestation (mean, 95th and 5th centiles)

of blood flows to and resistance to flow in the kidneys, other abdominal organs, femoral arteries (lower limbs) and placenta. Approximately 50% of blood flow in the descending thoracic aorta is distributed to the umbilical artery. With advancing gestation, the PI in the umbilical artery decreases, due to reduced resistance in the placental compartment, whereas, in the aorta, the PI remains constant. The absence of a change in PI suggests the presence of a compensatory vasoconstrictive mechanism in the other major branches of the aorta distribution, such as the extremities. The mean blood velocity

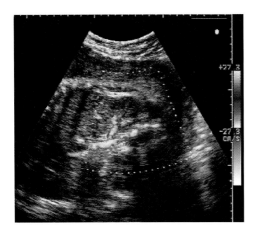 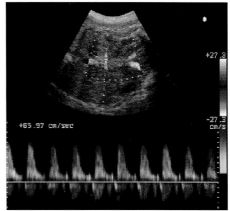

Figure 7 Parasagittal view of the fetal trunk with superimposed color Doppler showing the renal artery originating from the descending aorta (left). Flow velocity waveforms from the renal artery and vein at 32 weeks of gestation with physiologically absent end-diastolic velocities (right)

increases with gestation up to 32 weeks and then remains constant up to 40 weeks, when there is a small fall (Figure 6)[15].

Renal artery

Color Doppler allows easy identification in a longitudinal view of the fetal renal artery from its origin as a lateral branch of the abdominal aorta to the hilus of the kidney (Figure 7). Diastolic velocities may be physiologically absent until 34 weeks, and then increase significantly with advancing gestation. The PI decreases linearly with gestation, indicating a fall in impedance to flow, and presumably an increase in renal perfusion[16,17]. This may offer an explanation for the increase of fetal urine production that occurs with advancing gestation[18].

Cerebral arteries

With the color Doppler technique, it is possible to investigate the main cerebral arteries such as the internal carotid artery, the middle cerebral artery, and the anterior and the posterior cerebral arteries and to evaluate the vascular resistances in different areas supplied by these vessels.

A transverse view of the fetal brain is obtained at the level of the biparietal diameter. The transducer is then moved towards the base of the skull at the level of the lesser wing of the sphenoid bone. Using color flow imaging, the middle cerebral artery can be seen as a major lateral branch of the circle of Willis, running anterolaterally at the borderline

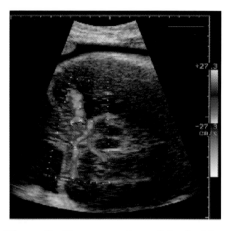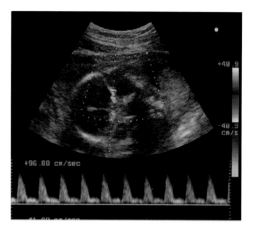

Figure 8 Transverse view of the fetal head with superimposed color Doppler showing the circle of Willis (left). Flow velocity waveforms from the middle cerebral artery at 32 weeks of gestation (right)

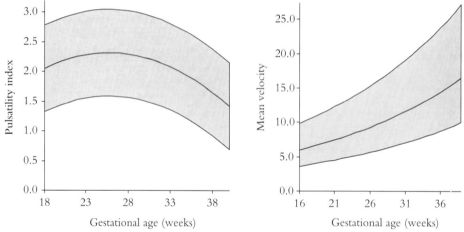

Figure 9 Pulsatility index (left) and mean blood velocity (right) in the fetal middle cerebral artery with gestation (mean, 95th and 5th centiles)

between the anterior and the middle cerebral fossae (Figure 8). The pulsed Doppler sample gate is then placed on the middle portion of this vessel to obtain flow velocity waveforms. Due to the course of this blood vessel, it is almost always possible to obtain an angle of insonation which is less than 10°. During the studies, care should be taken to apply minimal pressure to the maternal abdomen with the transducer, as fetal head compression is associated with alterations of intracranial arterial waveforms[19].

In healthy fetuses, impedance to flow in the fetal aorta does not change with gestation during the second and early third trimesters of pregnancy, but it subsequently

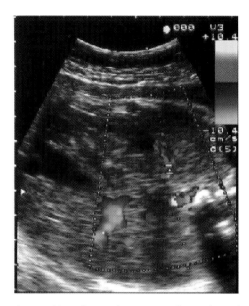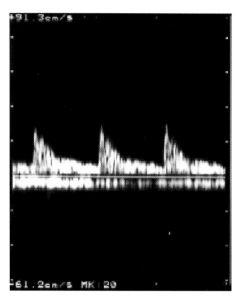

Figure 10 Flow velocity waveforms from the fetal splenic artery at 32 weeks of gestation in a fetus with ascites

decreases (Figure 9)[15,20–22]. The PI is significantly higher in the middle cerebral artery than in the internal carotid artery or in the anterior and posterior cerebral arteries. It is, therefore, important to know exactly which cerebral vessel is sampled during a Doppler examination, as a PI value that might be normal for the internal carotid artery may be abnormal for the middle cerebral artery. The use of color Doppler greatly improves the identification of the cerebral vessels, thus limiting the possibility of sampling errors. The blood velocity increases with advancing gestation, and this increase is significantly associated with the decrease in PI (Figure 9).

Other arterial vessels

Improvements in flow detection with the new generation of color Doppler equipment have made it possible to visualize and record velocity waveforms from several fetal arterial vessels, including those to the extremities (femoral, tibial and brachial arteries), adrenal, splenic (Figure 10), mesenteric, lung, and coronary vessels. Although study of these vessels has helped to improve our knowledge of fetal hemodynamics, there is no evidence at present to support their use in clinical practice.

FETAL CARDIAC FLOW

Examination of the fetal heart using Doppler ultrasound is achieved similarly to the examination in gray-scale mode. Several planes including the abdominal view,

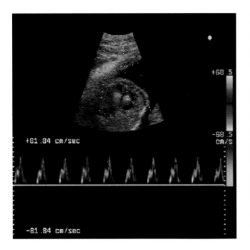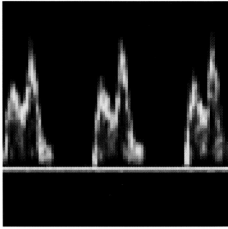

Figure 11   Flow velocity waveform across the tricuspid valve at 28 weeks of gestation. Note the absence of flow during systole and the presence of two peaks during diastole (E–wave = early ventricular filling and A–wave = atrial ventricular filling)

four-chamber, five-chamber, short-axis and three-vessel views have to be assessed in order to get spatial information on different cardiac chambers and vessels, as well as their connections to each other. The difference in the application of color Doppler is the insonation angle, which should be as small as possible to permit optimal visualization of flow.

In the abdominal plane, the position of the aorta and inferior vena cava are first checked as well as the correct connection of the vein to the right atrium. Pulsed Doppler sampling from the interior vena cava, the ductus venosus or the hepatic veins can be achieved in longitudinal planes. The next plane, the four-chamber view, is considered as the most important, since it allows an easy detection of numerous severe heart defects. Using color Doppler in an apical or basal approach, the diastolic perfusion across the atrioventricular valves can be assessed (Figure 11). The separate perfusion of both inflow tracts is characteristic. The sampling of diastolic flow using pulsed Doppler will show the typical biphasic shape of diastolic flow velocity waveform with an early peak diastolic velocity (E) and a second peak during atrial contraction (A–wave). E is smaller than A and the E/A ratio increases during pregnancy toward 1, to be inversed after birth (Figure 12). In this plane, regurgitations of the atrioventricular valves, which are more frequent at the tricuspid valve, are easily detected during systole using color Doppler.

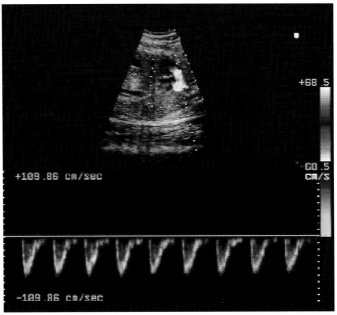

Figure 14 Flow velocity waveform from the pulmonary artery at 32 weeks of gestation

according to the site of sampling and there is a progressive increase in the diastolic component in the more distal vessels[40,41] (Figure 14). Their analysis may be used to study the normal development of lung circulation.

Ductus arteriosus

Ductal velocity waveforms are recorded from a short-axis view showing the ductal arch and are characterized by a continuous forward flow through the entire cardiac cycle[42]. The parameter most commonly analyzed is the PV during systole or, similarly to peripheral vessels, the pulsatility index [PI = (systolic velocity − diastolic velocity)/ time averaged maximum velocity][42,43].

Errors in Doppler blood flow velocity waveforms

A major concern in obtaining absolute measurements of velocities or flow is their reproducibility. To obtain reliable recordings, it is particularly important to minimize the angle of insonation, to verify in real-time and color flow imaging the correct position of the sample volume before and after each Doppler recording, and to limit the recordings to periods of fetal rest and apnea, as behavioral states greatly influence the recordings[44,45]. In these conditions, it is necessary to select a series of at least five consecutive velocity waveforms characterized by uniform morphology and high signal to noise ratio before performing the measurements. Using this technique of recording and analysis, it is possible to achieve a coefficient of variation below 10% for all the echocardiographic indices with the exception of those needing the valve dimensions[46–48].

Normal ranges of Doppler echocardiographic indices

It is possible to record cardiac flow velocity waveforms from as early as 8 weeks of gestation by transvaginal color Doppler[49,50]. In early pregnancy (8–20 weeks), there are major changes at all cardiac levels. The E/A ratio at both atrioventricular levels increases[49–51]. PV and TVI in outflow tracts increase and this is particularly evident at the level of the pulmonary valve[49]. These changes suggest a rapid development of ventricular compliance and a shift of cardiac output towards the right ventricle; this shift is probably secondary to decreased right ventricle afterload which, in turn, is due to the fall in placental resistance.

At the level of the atrioventricular valves, the E/A ratios increase[52,53], while PV values linearly increase at the level of both pulmonary and aortic valves[54]. Small changes are present in TPV values during gestation[55]. TPV values at the level of the pulmonary valve are lower than at aortic level, suggesting a slightly higher blood pressure in the pulmonary artery than in the ascending aorta[56]. Quantitative measurements have shown that the right cardiac output (RCO) is higher than the left cardiac output (LCO) and that, from 20 weeks onwards, the RCO to LCO ratio remains constant, with a mean value of 1.3[57,58]. This value is lower than that reported in fetal sheep (RCO/LCO = 1.8), and this difference may be explained by the higher brain weight in humans which necessitates an increase in left cardiac output[59].

In normal fetuses, VEF exponentially increases with advancing gestation, both at the level of the right and left ventricles[27]. No significant differences are present between right and left VEF values and the ratio between right and left VEF values remains stable with advancing gestation (mean value = 1.09)[27].

Ductal PV increases linearly with gestation and its values represent the highest velocity in the fetal circulation occurring in normal conditions while the PI is constant[42,43]. Values of systolic velocity above 140 cm/s, in conjunction with a diastolic velocity greater than 35 cm/s or a PI of less than 1.9, are considered to be an expression of ductal constriction[42].

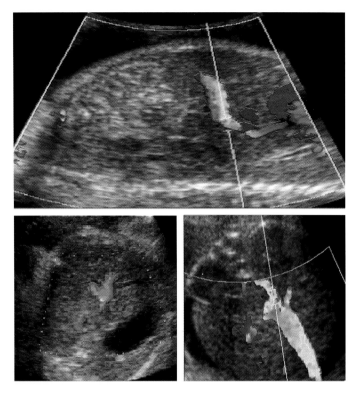

Figure 15 Sagittal view of the fetal thorax and abdomen showing the ductus venosus (top). Transverse section of the fetal abdomen showing the ductus venosus originating from the umbilical vein (bottom, left) and transverse oblique view demonstrating the aliasing effect (bottom, right)

FETAL VENOUS FLOW

Anatomy

The fetal liver with its venous vasculature – umbilical and portal veins, ductus venosus and hepatic veins – and the inferior vena cava are the main areas of interest in the investigation of venous blood return to the fetal heart. The intra-abdominal part of the umbilical vein ascends relatively steeply from the cord insertion in the inferior part of the falciform ligament. Then the vessel continues in a more horizontal and posterior direction and turns to the right to the confluence with the transverse part of the left portal vein, which joins the right portal vein with its division into an anterior and a posterior branch.

The ductus venosus originates from the umbilical vein before it turns to the right (Figure 15). The diameter of the ductus venosus measures approximately one-third of

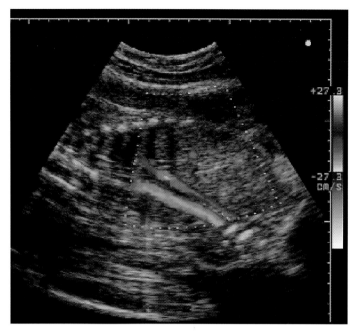

Figure 16 Parasagittal view of the fetal trunk with superimposed color Doppler showing the descending aorta (blue) and the inferior vena cava (red)

that of the umbilical vein. It courses posteriorly and in a cephalad direction, with increasing steepness in the same sagittal plane as the original direction of the umbilical vein, and enters the inferior vena cava in a venous vestibulum just below the diaphragm. The three (left, middle, and right) hepatic veins reach the inferior vena cava in the same funnel-like structure[60].

The ductus venosus can be visualized in its full length in a mid-sagittal longitudinal section of the fetal trunk (Figure 15). In an oblique transverse section through the upper abdomen, its origin from the umbilical vein can be found where color Doppler indicates high velocities compared to the umbilical vein, and sometimes this produces an aliasing effect (Figure 15). The blood flow velocity accelerates due to the narrow lumen of the ductus venosus, the maximum inner width of the narrowest portion being 2 mm[61]. The best ultrasound plane to depict the inferior vena cava is a longitudinal or coronal one, where it runs anterior, to the right of and nearly parallel to the descending aorta (Figure 16). The hepatic veins can be visualized, either in a transverse section through the upper abdomen or in a sagittal–coronal section through the appropriate lobe of the liver.

Physiology

The ductus venosus plays a central role in the return of venous blood from the placenta. Well-oxygenated blood flows via this shunt directly towards the heart. Approximately 40% of umbilical vein blood enters the ductus venosus and accounts for 98% of blood flow through the ductus venosus, because portal blood is directed almost exclusively to the right lobe of the liver[62]. Oxygen saturation is higher in the left hepatic vein compared to the right hepatic vein. This is due to the fact that the left lobe of the liver is supplied by branches from the umbilical vein.

Animal studies have shown that there is a streamlining of blood flow within the thoracic inferior vena cava[63]. Blood from the ductus venosus and the left hepatic vein flows in the dorsal and leftward part, whereas blood from the distal inferior vena cava and the right lobe of the liver flows in the ventral and rightward part of the inferior vena cava. The ventral and rightward stream, together with blood from the superior vena cava, is directed towards the right atrium and through the tricuspid valve into the right ventricle. From there the blood is ejected into the main pulmonary artery and most of it is shunted through the ductus arteriosus into the descending aorta. The dorsal and leftward stream is directed towards the foramen ovale, thereby delivering well-oxygenated blood directly to the left heart and from there via the ascending aorta to the myocardium and the brain. In sheep, the two bloodstreams show different flow velocities, with the higher velocity found in the stream that originates from the ductus venosus[64]. Color Doppler studies in human fetuses confirm these findings. The crista dividens, which forms the upper edge of the foramen ovale, separates the two pathways, and the blood delivered to the left atrium circumvents the right atrium[65].

The typical waveform for blood flow in venous vessels consists of three phases (Figure 17). The highest pressure gradient between the venous vessels and the right atrium occurs during ventricular systole (S), which results in the highest blood flow velocities towards the fetal heart during that part of the cardiac cycle. Early diastole (D), with the opening of the atrioventricular valves and passive early filling of the ventricles (E-wave of the biphasic atrioventricular flow waveform), is associated with a second peak of forward flow. The nadir of flow velocities coincides with atrial contraction (a) during late diastole (A-wave of the atrioventricular flow waveform). During atrial contraction, the foramen ovale flap and the crista dividens meet, thereby preventing direct blood flow from the ductus venosus to the left atrium during that short period of closure of the foramen ovale.

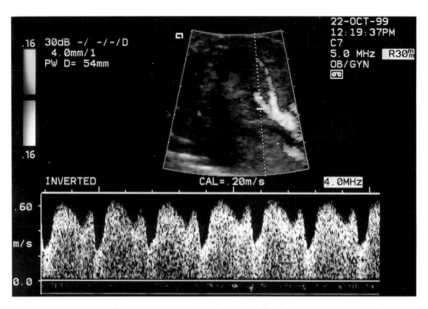

Figure 17 Normal flow velocity waveforms of the ductus venosus visualized in a sagittal section through the fetal abdomen. The first peak indicates systole, the second early diastole and the nadir of the waveform occurs during atrial contraction

Normal Doppler findings

The easiest vessel in which to investigate venous blood flow is the umbilical vein. Investigation of fetal venous umbilical blood flow by Doppler ultrasound was published in 1980 by Eik-Nes and colleagues[66] and in 1981 by Gill *et al.*[67]. They reported on mean volume flow in the intra-abdominal part of the umbilical vein, which averaged 110–120 ml/kg/min in uncomplicated third-trimester pregnancies. Continuous forward flow without pulsations is seen in most pregnancies after the first trimester. It is interesting that there seems to be an intrinsic inhibition of retrograde flow in the umbilical vein. This was concluded from a study comparing flow volume and velocity measurements of test fluid pumped through the cord under standardized conditions in antegrade and retrograde directions[68]. This was attributed to the orientation of the endothelial cells within the vessel wall.

In a study during early gestation, pulsations were always seen until 8 weeks and they progressively disappeared between 9 and 12 weeks[69]. Other investigators observed them up to 15 weeks and no relation between the pulsatility of venous waveforms and the descending aorta and umbilical artery could be established[70]. Changes in cardiac filling patterns were thought to be responsible for these findings. Other studies reported umbilical venous pulsations synchronous with the fetal heart rate in normal fetuses between 34 and 38 weeks[71]. They were present in 20% of measurements in a free-floating loop of the cord, in 33% of intra-abdominal umbilical venous measurements, and in 78% of waveforms from the umbilical sinus and left portal vein. These mild pulsations and the sinusoidal waveforms occurring during fetal breathing movements must be distinguished from severe pulsations showing a sharp decrease in blood flow, corresponding to the fetal heart rate in cases of fetal compromise.

There is an abrupt change in the blood flow waveforms at the origin of the ductus venosus from continuous to pulsatile flow and an approximately three- to four-fold increase in maximum velocities. An abrupt pressure drop is present at the entrance of the ductus venosus and there is a high-velocity jet from the inlet throughout the lower portion of the ductus, with a decrease of velocities toward its outlet due to its conicity[72]. Flow in the ductus venosus is directed toward the heart throughout the whole cycle. Even in early pregnancy, there is no retrograde flow during atrial contraction (Figure 18)[73]. The high velocities probably support the preferential direction of blood flow towards the foramen ovale, and avoid mixing with blood with lower oxygen saturation from the inferior vena cava and right hepatic vein. The mean peak velocities increase from 65 cm/s at 18 weeks to 75 cm/s at term[61].

In contrast to the ductus venosus waveform, atrial contraction can cause absence or reversal of blood flow in the inferior vena cava and this is almost always the case in the hepatic veins (Figures 19 and 20). The percentage of reverse flow in the inferior vena

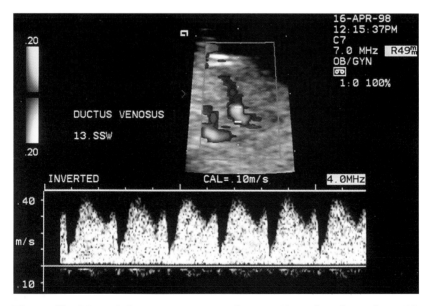

Figure 18 Normal ductus venosus waveform at 13 weeks of gestation with positive flow during atrial contraction

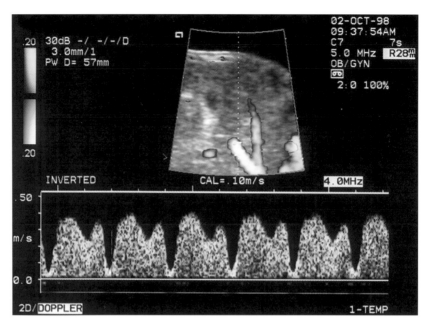

Figure 19 Ductus venosus flow velocity waveform with low but positive forward flow during atrial contraction. The blue signal cephalad from the ductus comes from the middle hepatic vein

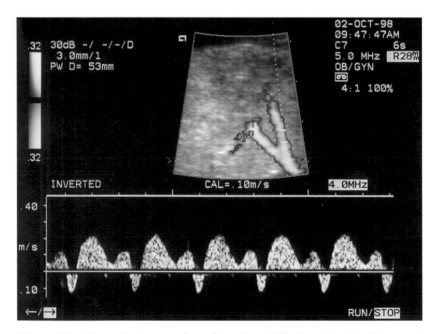

Figure 20 Flow velocity waveform from the middle hepatic vein. Compared to the ductus venosus (see Figure 19), the velocities are significantly lower and there is reversal of blood flow during atrial contraction

cava decreases with advancing gestational age. At 12–15 weeks, it is four- to five-fold of that seen near term. Studies attempting to describe the pulsatility of flow velocity wave-forms have used the S/D ratio in the inferior vena cava or ductus venosus[74–77], the preload index (a/S) in the inferior vena cava[78], and the resistance index [(S − a)/S] and the S/a ratio in the ductus venosus[79,80]. With one exception[76], no significant change with gestational age has been found for the S/D ratio. Similarly, no relationship has been found between the preload index and gestational age, which is inconsistent with the finding of a decrease in percentage of reverse flow with advancing gestation[78]. The ductus venosus index [(S − a)/S], which is equivalent to the resistance index, decreases significantly with gestational age[79]. This is in agreement with a decrease of the S/a ratio with gestational age, which also shows a significant relationship with the percentage of reverse flow in the inferior vena cava[80].

A study of blood flow in the ductus venosus, inferior vena cava and right hepatic vein in 143 normal fetuses during the second half of pregnancy established reference ranges for mean and maximum velocities and two indices for venous waveform analysis[81]. The first one was the peak velocity index [(S − a)/D] and the second one the equivalent to the PI [(S − a)/time-averaged maximum velocity]. Mean and peak blood velocities increased, whereas the indices decreased with advancing gestation (Figure 21). Velocities were highest in the ductus venosus and lowest in the right hepatic vein, whereas the lowest indices were found in the ductus venosus and highest indices in the right hepatic vein. The finding that the degree of pulsatility decreases with gestation is consistent with a decrease in cardiac afterload due to a decrease in placental resistance, and may also reflect increased ventricular compliance

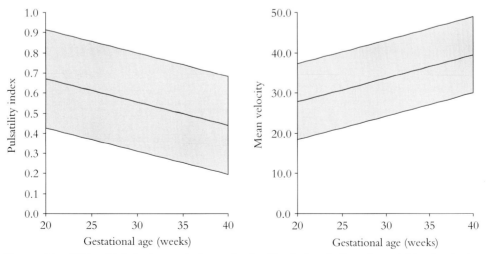

Figure 21 PIV, which is the equivalent of pulsatility index (left) and mean blood velocity (right) in the ductus venosus with gestation (mean, 95th and 5th centiles)

and maturation of cardiac function. A decrease in end-diastolic ventricular pressure causes an increase in venous blood flow velocity towards the heart during atrial contraction.

The sampling site is of crucial importance in venous Doppler studies. Velocities at the inlet of the ductus venosus, immediately above the umbilical vein, are higher than at the outlet into the inferior vena cava and the sampling site should be standardized at the inlet[82]. There are relatively wide limits of agreement for intraobserver variation for velocity measurements. Inferior vena cava signals at the entrance to the right atrium show a large standard deviation for various waveform parameters[74]. To avoid a mixture of overlapping signals from different bloodstreams, flow velocity waveforms from the inferior vena cava should be obtained more distally. The highest reproducibility of inferior vena cava waveforms is achieved by placing the sample volume between the entrance of the renal vein and the ductus venosus[83].

Generally, flow volume measurements and absolute velocity measurements seem to have considerably higher inaccuracies and intra-patient variations compared to velocity ratios. This is due to problems caused by a high or unreliable angle of insonation and the fact that vessel diameter measurements are very vulnerable to errors. Ratios and indices of velocities, on the other hand, are to a large extent independent of the angle of insonation. Furthermore, fetal behavioral states have to be taken into account when measuring blood flow velocities in the ductus venosus. A 30% decrease of velocities was found during fetal behavioral state 1F compared to 2F, but no change in S/D ratio[84].

Waveforms of the ductus venosus with very little or even without pulsatility seem to be normal variants. They were found in 3% of measurements in a longitudinal study of normal pregnancies[82]. There are conflicting reports on the existence of a sphincter regulating blood flow through the ductus venosus. Autonomous innervation may have an influence on ductal blood flow, but it is questionable whether there is an isolated muscular structure functioning as a sphincter. Apparent ductus venosus dilatation has been reported in two cases with growth-restricted fetuses, causing modifications of flow velocity waveforms with a reduction of velocities during atrial contraction and, consequently, an increase in pulsatility[85]. These findings were confirmed in a simulation of ductal dilatation by means of a mathematical model.

During Doppler studies of the fetal circulation, it is essential to avoid measurements during fetal breathing movements. This is well described for the arterial side but it is even more important for venous flow, because the changes in intrathoracic pressure during breathing movements have a profound influence on flow velocity waveforms. A raised abdomino–thoracic pressure gradient seems to be responsible for this phenomenon. By applying the Bernoulli equation, the pressure gradient across the ductus venosus ranges between 0 and 3 mmHg during the heart cycle, but increases to 22 mmHg during fetal inspiratory movements[86]. As the shape of velocity waveforms during breathing movements shows persistent changes, velocity ratios or indices should only be calculated during fetal apnea.

On the other hand, comparison between umbilical arterial and venous waveforms during fetal breathing movements offers an interesting model to investigate the interdependence between fetal cardiovascular and placental blood flow[87]. Variation in umbilical venous velocity may alter placental filling and thereby affect umbilical arterial diastolic velocity. It may also alter ventricular filling and thereby affect umbilical arterial systolic velocity through the Frank–Starling mechanism, which results in limited changes in stroke volume. Therefore, changes in velocity of venous blood flow returning to the heart have an influence on velocities of arterial blood flow returning to the placenta and *vice versa*. In other words, cardiac preload influences afterload and is influenced by afterload itself.

Recent studies have investigated the venous circulation of the fetal brain and various sinuses[88,89]. The increase of flow velocities and decrease of pulsatility with gestational age and the increase of the pulsatility of waveforms from the periphery toward the proximal portion of the venous vasculature is in accordance with findings in precardial venous vessels.

REFERENCES

1. Giles WB, Trudinger BJ, Paimer AA. Umbilical cord whole blood viscosity and the umbilical artery flow velocity time waveforms: a correlation. *Br J Obstet Gynaecol* 1986;93:466
2. Boyd JD, Hamilton WJ. *The Human Placenta*. Cambridge: Heffer & Sons, 1970:207–74
3. Ramsey EM, Corner GW, Donner MW. Serial and cineradioangiographic visualization of maternal circulation in the primate (hemochorial) placenta. *Am J Obstet Gynecol* 1963;86:213–25
4. Brosens I, Robertson WB, Dixon HG. The physiological response of the vessels of the placental bed to normal pregnancy. *J Pathol Bacteriol* 1967;93:569–79
5. Pijnenborg R, Bland JM, Robertson WB, Brosens I. Uteroplacental arterial changes related to interstitial trophoblast migration in early human pregnancy. *Placenta* 1983;4:387–414
6. Assali NS, Rauramo L, Peltonen T. Measurement of uterine blood flow and uterine metabolism. VIII. Uterine and fetal blood flow and oxygen consumption in early human pregnancy. *Am J Obstet Gynecol* 1960;79:86–98
7. Browne JCM, Veall N. The maternal placental blood flow in normotensive and hypertensive women. *J Obstet Gynaecol Br Empire* 1953;60:141–7
8. Campbell S, Diaz-Recasens J, Griffin DR, Cohen-Overbeek TE, Pearce JM, Willson K, Teague MJ. New Doppler technique for assessing uteroplacental blood inflow. *Lancet* 1983;i:675–7

9. Trudinger BJ, Giles WB, Cook CM. Uteroplacental blood flow velocity-time waveforms in normal and complicated pregnancy. *Br J Obstet Gynaecol* 1985;92:39–45

10. Schulman H, Fleischer A, Farmakides G, Bracero L, Rochelson B, Grunfeld L. Development of uterine artery compliance in pregnancy as detected by Doppler ultrasound. *Am J Obstet Gynecol* 1986;155:1031–6

11. Bewley S, Campbell S, Cooper D. Uteroplacental Doppler flow velocity waveforms in the second trimester. A complex circulation. *Br J Obstet Gynaecol* 1989;96:1040–6

12. Arduini D, Rizzo G, Boccolini MR, Romanini C, Mancuso S. Functional assessment of utero-placental and fetal circulations by means of color Doppler ultrasonography. *J Ultrasound Med* 1990;9:249–53

13. Maulik D, Yarlagadda P, Downing G. Doppler velocimetry in obstetrics. *Obstet Gynecol Clin North Am* 1990;17:163–86

14. Maulik D. Basic principles of Doppler ultrasound as applied in obstetrics. *Clin Obstet Gynecol* 1989;32:628–44

15. Bilardo CM, Campbell S, Nicolaides KH. Mean blood velocities and flow impedance in the fetal descending thoracic aortic and common carotid artery in normal pregnancy. *Early Hum Dev* 1988;18:213–21

16. Vyas S, Nicolaides KH, Campbell S. Renal artery flow-velocity waveforms in normal and hypoxemic fetuses. *Am J Obstet Gynecol* 1989;161:168–72

17. Hecher K, Spernol R, Szalay S. Doppler blood flow velocity waveforms in the fetal renal artery. *Arch Gynecol Obstet* 1989;246:133–7

18. Rabinowitz R, Peters MT, Vyas S, Campbell S, Nicolaides KH. Measurement of fetal urine production in normal pregnancy by real-time ultrasonography. *Am J Obstet Gynecol* 1989;161:1264–6

19. Vyas S, Campbell S, Bower S, Nicolaides KH. Maternal abdominal pressure alters fetal cerebral blood flow. *Br J Obstet Gynaecol* 1990;97:740–2

20. Kirkinen P, Muller R, Huch R, Huch A. Blood flow velocity waveforms in human fetal intra-cranial arteries. *Obstet Gynecol* 1987,70:617–21

21. van den Wiingaard JAGW, Groenenberg IAL, Wiadimiroff JW, Hop WCJ. Cerebral Doppler ultrasound in the human fetus. *Br J Obstet Gynaecol* 1989;96:845–9

22. Vyas S, Nicolaides KH, Bower S, Campbell S. Middle cerebral artery flow velocity waveforms in fetal hypoxaemia. *Br J Obstet Gynaecol* 1990;97:797–803

23. Burns PN. Doppler flow estimations in the fetal and maternal circulations: principles, techniques and some limitations. In Maulik D, McNellis D, eds. *Doppler Ultrasound Measurement of Maternal-Fetal Hemodynamics*. Ithaca, New York, USA: Perinatology Press, 1987:43–78

24. Rizzo G, Arduini D, Romanini C. Doppler echocardiographic assessment of fetal cardiac function. *Ultrasound Obstet Gynecol* 1992;2:434–45

25. Comstock CH, Riggs T, Lee W, Kirk J. Pulmonary to aorta diameter ratio in the normal and abnormal fetal heart. *Am J Obstet Gynecol* 1991;165:1038–43

26. St John Sutton M, Gill T, Plappert T, Saltzman DH, Doubilet P. Assessment of right and left ventricular function in term of force development with gestational age in the normal human fetus. *Br Heart J* 1991;61:285–9

27. Rizzo G, Capponi A, Rinaldo D, Arduini D, Romanini C. Ventricular ejection force in growth-retarded fetuses. *Ultrasound Obstet Gynecol* 1995;5:247–52

28. Isaaz K, Ethevenot G, Admant P, Brembilla B, Pernot C. A new Doppler method of assessing left ventricular ejection force in chronic congestive heart failure. *Am J Cardiol* 1989; 64:81–7

29. Stottard MF, Pearson AC, Kern MJ, Ratcliff J, Mrosek DG, Labovitz AJ. Influence of alteration in preload of left ventricular diastolic filling as assessed by Doppler echocardiography in humans. *Circulation* 1989;79:1226–36

30. Gardin JM. Doppler measurements of aortic blood velocity and acceleration: load-independent indexes of left ventricular performance. *Am J Cardiol* 1989;64:935–6

31. Bedotto JB, Eichorn EJ, Grayburn PA. Effects of left ventricular preload and afterload on ascending aortic blood velocity and acceleration in coronaric artery disease. *Am J Cardiol* 1989:64:856–9

32. Brownwall E, Ross J, Sonnenblick EH. *Mechanism of Contraction in the Normal and Failing Heart*, 2nd edn. Boston: Little Brown, 1976, 92–129

33. Takaneka K, Dabestani A, Gardin JM, Russel D, Clark S, Allfie A, Henry WL. Left ventricular filling in hypertrophic cardiomyopathy: a pulsed Doppler echocardiographic study. *J Am Coll Cardiol* 1986;7:1263–71

34. Kenny J, Plappert T, Doubilet P, Saltzam D, St John Sutton MG. Effects of heart rate on ventricular size, stroke volume and output in the normal human fetus: a prospective Doppler echocardiographic study. *Circulation* 1987;76:52–8

35. Labovitz AJ, Pearson C. Evaluation of left ventricular diastolic function: clinical relevance and recent Doppler echocardiographic insights. *Am Heart J* 1987;114:836–51

36. Kitabatake A, Inoue M, Asao M, *et al.* Noninvasive evaluation of pulmonary hypertension by a pulsed Doppler technique. *Circulation* 1983;68:302–9

37. Baschat AA, Gembruch U, Reiss I, Gortner L, Diedrich K. Demonstration of fetal coronary blood flow by Doppler ultrasound in relation to arterial and venous flow velocity waveforms and perinatal outcome. The heart sparing effect. *Ultrasound Obstet Gynecol* 1997;9:162–72

38. Laudy JAM, De Riddler MA, Wladimiroff J. Doppler velocimetry in branch pulmonary arteries of normal human fetuses during the second half of pregnancy. *Pediatr Res* 1997;41:897–901

39. Rasanen J, Huhta JC, Weiner S, Wood DC, Ludormisky A. Fetal branch pulmonary arterial vascular impedance during the second half of pregnancy. *Am J Obstet Gynecol* 1996;174:1441–9

40. Rizzo G, Capponi A, Chaoui R, Taddei F, Arduini D, Romanini C. Blood flow velocity waveforms from peripheral pulmonary arteries in normally grown and growth-retarded fetuses. *Ultrasound Obstet Gynecol* 1996;8:87–92

41. Chaoui R, Taddei F, Rizzo G, Bast C, Lenz F, Bollmann R. Doppler echocardiography of the main stems of the pulmonary arteries in the normal human fetus. *Ultrasound Obstet Gynecol* 1998;11: 173–9

42. Huhta JC, Moise KJ, Fisher DJ, Sharif DF, Wasserstrum N, Martin C. Detection and quantitation of constriction of the fetal ductus arteriosus by Doppler echocardiography. *Circulation* 1987;75, 406–12

43. Van de Mooren K, Barendregt LG, Wladimiroff J. Flow velocity waveforms in the human fetal ductus arteriosus during the normal second trimester of pregnancy. *Pediatr Res* 1991;30:487–90

44. Rizzo G, Arduini D, Valensise H, Romanini C. Effects of behavioural states on cardiac output in the healthy human fetus at 36–38 weeks of gestation. *Early Hum Dev* 1990;23:109–15

45. Huisman TW, Brezinka C, Stewart PA, Stijen T, Wladimiroff JW. Ductus venosus flow velocity waveforms in relation to fetal behavioural states. *Br J Obstet Gynaecol* 1994;101:220–4

46. Groenenberg IAL, Hop WCJ, Wladimiroff JW. Doppler flow velocity waveforms in the fetal cardiac outflow tract; reproducibility of waveform recording and analysis. *Ultrasound Med Biol* 1991; 17:583–7

47. Al-Ghazali W, Chita SK, Chapman MG, Allan LD. Evidence of redistribution of cardiac output in asymmetrical growth retardation. *Br J Obstet Gynaecol* 1989; 96:697–704

48. Reed KL, Meijboom EJ, Sahn DJ, Scagnelli SA, Valdes-Cruz LM, Skenker L. Cardiac Doppler flow velocities in human fetuses. *Circulation* 1986;73:41–56

49. Rizzo G, Arduini D, Romanini C. Fetal cardiac and extra-cardiac circulation in early gestation. *J Maternal-Fetal Invest* 1991;1:73–8

50. van Splunder P, Stijnen T, Wladimiroff JW. Fetal atrioventricular flow-velocity waveforms and their relationship to arterial and venous flow velocity waveforms at 8 to 20 weeks of gestation. *Circulation* 1996;94:1372–8

51. Wladimiroff JW, Huisman TWA, Stewart PA, Stijnen Th. Normal fetal Doppler inferior vena cava, transtricuspid and umbilical artery flow velocity waveforms between 11 and 16 weeks' gestation. *Am J Obstet Gynecol* 1992;166:46–9

52. Reed KL, Sahn DJ, Scagnelli S, Anderson CF, Shenker L. Doppler echocardiographic studies of diastolic function in the human fetal heart: changes during gestation. *J Am Coll Cardiol* 1986;8: 391–5

53. Rizzo G, Arduini D, Romanini C, Mancuso S. Doppler echocardiographic assessment of atrioventricular velocity waveforms in normal and small for gestational age fetuses. *Br J Obstet Gynaecol* 1988;95:65–9

54. Kenny JF, Plappert T, Saltzman DH, Cartire M, Zollars L, Leatherman GF, St John Sutton MG. Changes in intracardiac blood flow velocities and right and left ventricular stroke volumes with gestational age in the normal human fetus: a prospective Doppler echocardiographic study. *Circulation* 1986;74:1208–16

55. Rizzo G, Arduini D, Romanini C, Mancuso S. Doppler echocardiographic evaluation of time to peak velocity in the aorta and pulmonary artery of small for gestational age fetuses. *Br J Obstet Gynaecol* 1990;97:603–7

56. Machado MVL, Chita SC, Allan LD. Acceleration time in the aorta and pulmonary artery measured by Doppler echocardiography in the midtrimester normal human fetus. *Br Heart J* 1987;58:15–18

57. Allan LD, Chita SK, Al-Ghazali W, Crawford DC, Tynan M. Doppler echocardiographic evaluation of the normal human fetal heart. *Br Heart J* 1987;57:528–33

58. De Smedt MCH, Visser GHA, Meijboom EJ. Fetal cardiac output estimated by Doppler echocardiography during mid- and late gestation. *Am J Cardiol* 1987;60:338–42

59. Rizzo G, Arduini D. Cardiac output in anencephalic fetuses. *Gynecol Obstet Invest* 1991;32:33–5

60. Huisman TWA, Gittenberger-De Groot AC, Wladimiroff JW. Recognition of a fetal subdiaphragmatic venous vestibulum essential for fetal venous Doppler assessment. *Pediatr Res* 1992;32:338–41

61. Kiserud T, Eik-Nes SH, Blaas HGK, Hellevik LR. Ultrasonographic velocimetry of the fetal ductus venosus. *Lancet* 1991;338:1412–14

62. Edelstone DI, Rudolph AM, Heymann MA. Liver and ductus venosus blood flows in fetal lambs *in utero*. *Circ Res* 1978;42:426–33

63. Edelstone DI, Rudolph AM. Preferential streaming of ductus venosus blood to the brain and heart in fetal lambs. *Am J Physiol* 1979;237:H724–9

64. Schmidt KG, Silverman NH, Rudolph AM. Assessment of flow events at the ductus venosus–inferior vena cava junction and at the foramen ovale in fetal sheep by use of multimodal ultrasound. *Circulation* 1996;93:826–33

65. Kiserud T, Eik-Nes SH, Blaas HG, Hellevik LR. Foramen ovale: an ultrasonographic study of its relation to the inferior vena cava, ductus venosus and hepatic veins. *Ultrasound Obstet Gynecol* 1992;2:389–96

66. Eik-Nes SH, Brubakk AO, Ulstein MK. Measurement of human fetal blood flow. *Br Med J* 1980; 280:283–4

67. Gill RW, Trudinger BJ, Garrett WJ, Kossoff G, Warren, PS. Fetal umbilical venous flow measured *in utero* by pulsed Doppler and B-mode ultrasound. I. Normal pregnancies. *Am J Obstet Gynecol* 1981;139:720–5

68. Potter PL. In vitro demonstration of inhibition of retrograde flow in the human umbilical vein. *Ultrasound Obstet Gynecol* 1997;9:319–23

69. Rizzo G, Arduini D, Romanini C. Umbilical vein pulsations: a physiologic finding in early gestation. *Am J Obstet Gynecol* 1992;167:675–7

70. van Splunder P, Huisman TWA, de Ridder MAJ, Wladimiroff JW. Fetal venous and arterial flow velocity wave forms between eight and twenty weeks of gestation. *Pediatr Res* 1996;40:158–62

71. van Splunder IP, Huisman TWA, Stijnen T, Wladimiroff JW. Presence of pulsations and reproducibility of waveform recording in the umbilical and left portal vein in normal pregnancies. *Ultrasound Obstet Gynecol* 1994;4:49–53

72. Pennati G, Bellotti M, Ferrazzi E, Rigano S, Garberi A. Hemodynamic changes across the human ductus venosus: a comparison between clinical findings and mathematical calculations. *Ultrasound Obstet Gynecol* 1997;9:383–91

73. Huisman TWA, Stewart PA, Wladimiroff JW, Stijnen T. Flow velocity waveforms in the ductus venosus, umbilical vein and inferior vena cava in normal human fetuses at 12–15 weeks of gestation. *Ultrasound Med Biol* 1993;19:441–5

74. Huisman TWA, Stewart PA, Wladimiroff JW. Flow velocity waveforms in the fetal inferior vena cava during the second half of normal pregnancy. *Ultrasound Med Biol* 1991;17:679–82

75. Huisman TWA, Stewart PA, Wladimiroff JW. Ductus venosus blood flow velocity waveforms in the human fetus – a Doppler study. *Ultrasound Med Biol* 1992;18:33–7

76. Reed KL, Appleton CP, Anderson CF, Shenker L, Sahn DJ. Doppler studies of vena cava flows in human fetuses. Insights into normal and abnormal cardiac physiology. *Circulation* 1990;81:498–505

77. Rizzo G, Arduini D, Romanini C. Inferior vena cava flow velocity waveforms in appropriate- and small-for-gestational-age fetuses. *Am J Obstet Gynecol* 1992;166:1271–80

78. Kanzaki T, Chiba Y. Evaluation of the preload condition of the fetus by inferior vena caval blood flow pattern. *Fetal Diagn Ther* 1990;5:168–74

79. DeVore GR, Horenstein J. Ductus venosus index: a method for evaluating right ventricular preload in the second-trimester fetus. *Ultrasound Obstet Gynecol* 1993;3:338–42

80. Rizzo G, Capponi A, Arduini D, Romanini C. Ductus venosus velocity waveforms in appropriate and small for gestational age fetuses. *Early Hum Dev* 1994;39:15–26

81. Hecher K, Campbell S, Snijders R, Nicolaides K. Reference ranges for fetal venous and atrioventricular blood flow parameters. *Ultrasound Obstet Gynecol* 1994;4:381–90

82. Kiserud T, Eik-Nes SH, Hellevik LR, Blaas HG. Ductus venosus – a longitudinal Doppler velocimetric study of the human fetus. *J Matern Fetal Invest* 1992;2:5–11

83. Rizzo G, Arduini D, Caforio L, Romanini C. Effects of sampling sites on inferior vena cava flow velocity waveforms. *J Matern Fetal Invest* 1992;2:153–6

84. Huisman TWA, Brezinka C, Stewart PA, Stijnen T, Wladimiroff JW. Ductus venosus flow velocity waveforms in relation to fetal behavioural states. *Br J Obstet Gynaecol* 1994;101: 20–4

85. Bellotti M, Pennati G, Pardi G, Fumero R. Dilatation of the ductus venosus in human fetuses: ultrasonographic evidence and mathematical modeling. *Am J Physiol* 1998; 275:H1759–67

86. Kiserud T, Hellevik LR, Eik-Nes SH, Angelsen BAJ, Blaas HG. Estimation of the pressure gradient across the fetal ductus venosus based on Doppler velocimetry. *Ultrasound Med Biol* 1994;20:225–32

87. Indik J, Reed KL. Variation and correlation in human fetal umbilical Doppler velocities with fetal breathing: evidence of the cardiac–placental connection. *Am J Obstet Gynecol* 1990;163:1792–6

88. Laurichesse-Delmas H, Grimaud O, Moscoso G, Ville Y. Color Doppler study of the venous circulation in the fetal brain and hemodynamic study of the cerebral transverse sinus. *Ultrasound Obstet Gynecol* 1999;13:34–42

89. Pooh RK, Pooh KH, Nakagawa Y, Maeda K, Fukui R, Aono T. Transvaginal Doppler assessment of fetal intracranial venous flow. *Obstet Gynecol* 1999;93:697–701

4

Doppler studies in fetal hypoxemic hypoxia

FETAL OXYGENATION

Oxygenation is the process of transporting molecular oxygen from air to the tissues of the body. In the fetus, this involves, first, oxygen transfer across the placenta, second, reversible binding of oxygen to fetal hemoglobin and fetal blood flow, and, third, oxygen consumption for growth and metabolism.

Energy is derived from the combination of oxygen and glucose to form carbon dioxide and water. Removal of carbon dioxide and protection against acidosis is by the reverse of the mechanisms for oxygen delivery and is helped by the rapid diffusion, high solubility and volatility of this gas. In the adult, carbon dioxide is excreted in the lungs while bicarbonate and hydrogen ions are removed by the kidney. In the fetus, both these functions are carried out by the placenta. When there is inadequate oxygen supply, the Krebs cycle cannot operate and pyruvate is converted to lactic acid. This enters the blood, leading to systemic acidosis unless it is either metabolized or excreted.

The amount of oxygen bound to hemoglobin is not linearly related to oxygen tension (pO_2). Each type of hemoglobin has a characteristic oxygen dissociation curve which can be modified by environmental factors, such as pH and the concentration of 2,3-diphosphoglycerate (2,3-DPG). For example, when 2,3-DPG rises, in response to anemia or hypoxia, it binds to and stabilizes the deoxygenated form of hemoglobin, resulting in a shift of the oxygen dissociation curve to the right and therefore release of oxygen to the tissues. Although, *in vitro*, both adult (HbA) and fetal (HbF) hemoglobins have the same oxygen dissociation curves, human adult blood has a lower affinity for oxygen than fetal because of its greater binding of 2,3-DPG. The higher affinity of fetal blood helps placental transfer of oxygen. Furthermore, since the P_{50} of fetal blood is similar to the umbilical arterial pO_2, the fetus operates over the steepest part of the hemoglobin oxygen dissociation curve and, therefore, a relatively large amount of oxygen is released from the hemoglobin for a given drop in pO_2.

Normal fetal oxygenation

In normal fetuses, the blood oxygen tension is much lower than the maternal, and it has been suggested that this is due either to incomplete venous equilibration of uterine and umbilical circulations and/or to high placental oxygen consumption[1,2]. Studies in a variety of animals have also demonstrated that the umbilical venous blood pO_2 is less than half the maternal arterial pO_2 and this observation led to the concept of 'Mount Everest *in utero*'. However, the high affinity of fetal hemoglobin for oxygen, together with the high fetal cardiac output in relation to oxygen demand, compensates for the low fetal pO_2[3].

The umbilical venous and arterial pO_2 and pH decrease, while pCO_2 increases, with gestation[1,2]. The blood oxygen content increases with gestational age because of the rise in fetal hemoglobin concentration[2]. Fetal blood lactate concentration does not change with gestation and the values are similar to those in samples obtained at elective Cesarean section at term[2]. The umbilical venous concentration is higher than the umbilical arterial, suggesting that the normoxemic human fetus is, like the sheep fetus, a net consumer of lactate[4]. Furthermore, the concentration of lactate in umbilical cord blood is higher than in the maternal blood and the two are correlated significantly. This suggests a common source of lactate, which is likely to be the placenta.

Fetal hypoxia

Fetal hypoxia, oxygen deficiency in the tissues, of any cause leads to a conversion from aerobic to anaerobic metabolism, which produces less energy and more acid. If the oxygen supply is not restored, the fetus dies. Hypoxia may result from:

(1) Reduced placental perfusion with maternal blood and consequent decrease in fetal arterial blood oxygen content due to low pO_2 (hypoxemic hypoxia);

(2) Reduced arterial blood oxygen content due to low fetal hemoglobin concentration (anemic hypoxia);

(3) Reduced blood flow to the fetal tissues (ischemic hypoxia).

Hypoxemic hypoxia (uteroplacental insufficiency)

Small-for-gestational age fetuses may be constitutionally small, with no increased perinatal death or morbidity, or they may be growth-restricted due to either low growth potential, the result of genetic disease or environmental damage, or due to reduced placental perfusion and 'uteroplacental insufficiency'.

Analysis of samples obtained by cordocentesis has demonstrated that some small-for-gestation fetuses are hypoxemic, hypercapnic, hyperlacticemic and acidemic[2,5]. Furthermore, both respiratory and metabolic acidemia increase with hypoxemia. In umbilical venous blood, mild hypoxemia may be present in the absence of hypercapnia or acidemia. In severe uteroplacental insufficiency, the fetus cannot compensate hemodynamically and hypercapnia and acidemia increase exponentially[2]. The carbon dioxide accumulation is presumably the result of reduced exchange between the uteroplacental and fetal circulations due to reduced blood flow. The association between hypoxemia and hyperlacticemia supports the concept of reduced oxidative metabolism of lactate being the cause of hyperlacticemia, and, under these circumstances, the fetus appears to be a net producer of lactate. Hypoxemic growth-restricted fetuses also demonstrate a whole range of hematological and metabolic abnormalities, including erythroblastemia, thrombocytopenia, hypoglycemia, deficiency in essential amino acids, hypertriglyceridemia, hypoinsulinemia and hypothyroidism[5-10].

Cross-sectional studies in pregnancies with growth-restricted fetuses have shown that increased impedance to flow in the uterine and umbilical arteries is associated with fetal hypoxemia and acidemia[11,12]. These data support the findings from histopathological studies that, in some pregnancies with small-for-gestation fetuses, there are:

(1) Failure of the normal development of maternal placental arteries into low-resistance vessels and therefore reduced oxygen and nutrient supply to the intervillous space[13];

(2) Reduction in the number of placental terminal capillaries and small muscular arteries in the tertiary stem villi and therefore impaired maternal–fetal transfer[14].

Animal studies have demonstrated that, in fetal hypoxemia, there is a redistribution in blood flow, with increased blood supply to the brain, heart and adrenals and a simultaneous reduction in the perfusion of the carcase, gut and kidneys[15]. Doppler ultrasound has enabled the non-invasive confirmation of the so-called 'brain-sparing' effect in human fetuses.

PATHOLOGICAL FINDINGS IN PRE-ECLAMPSIA AND INTRAUTERINE GROWTH RESTRICTION

Pre-eclampsia and intrauterine growth restriction are associated with an inadequate quality and quantity of the maternal vascular response to placentation. In both conditions, there are characteristic pathological findings in the placental bed. Brosens *et al.* examined placental bed biopsies from pregnancies complicated by pre-eclampsia and reported absence of physiological changes in the spiral arteries beyond the decidual–myometrial junction in more than 80% of the cases[13]. Robertson *et al.* examined placental bed biopsies from hypertensive women and found a difference between the lesions seen in women with pre-eclampsia and those with essential hypertension[16]. In pre-eclampsia, there was a necrotizing lesion with foam cells in the wall of the basal and spiral arteries, which was referred to as 'acute atherosis'. In essential hypertension, there were hyperplastic lesions in the basal and spiral arteries.

Sheppard and Bonnar reported that, in pregnancies with intrauterine growth restriction (irrespective of whether there is coexistent pre-eclampsia or not), there are atheromatous-like lesions that completely or partially occlude the spiral arteries; these changes are not present in pregnancies with pre-eclampsia in the absence of intrauterine growth restriction[17]. In contrast, Brosens *et al.* reported lack of physiological changes in all cases of pre-eclampsia, irrespective of the birth weight, and in most cases of intrauterine growth restriction; however, acute atherosis was found only in pre-eclampsia[18]. Khong *et al.* reviewed some of the archived biopsies of Brosens *et al.*[18,19]. They assessed the proportion of spiral arteries converted to uteroplacental arteries. In all cases of pre-eclampsia and in two-thirds of those with intrauterine growth restriction (defined as birth weight < 10th centile), there was no evidence of physiological change in the myometrial segments. Furthermore, complete absence of physiological change throughout the entire length of some spiral arteries was seen in approximately half the cases of pre-eclampsia and intrauterine growth restriction.

DOPPLER STUDIES

Uterine arteries

In pregnancies complicated by pre-eclampsia and/or intrauterine growth restriction, impedance to flow in the uterine arteries is increased (Figure 1). Studies in women with hypertensive disease of pregnancy have reported that, in those with increased impedance (increased resistance index or the presence of an early diastolic notch), compared to hypertensive women with normal flow velocity waveforms, there is a higher incidence of pre-eclampsia, intrauterine growth restriction, emergency Cesarean delivery, placental abruption, shorter duration of pregnancy and poorer neonatal outcome[20-23].

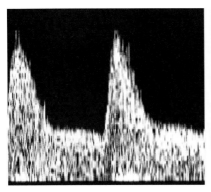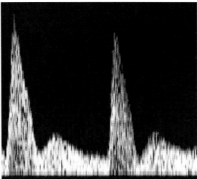

Figure 1 Normal (left) and abnormal (right) flow velocity waveforms from the uterine arteries at 24 weeks of gestation

Umbilical arteries

Pathological studies have demonstrated that increased impedance in the umbilical arteries becomes evident only when at least 60% of the placental vascular bed is obliterated[14]. In pregnancies with reversed or absent end–diastolic frequencies in the umbilical artery, compared to those with normal flow, mean placental weight is reduced and the cross-sectional diameter of terminal villi is shorter[24]. In pregnancies with fetal growth restriction, those with absent end–diastolic frequencies, compared to those with normal Doppler, have more fetal stem vessels with medial hyperplasia and luminal obliteration, and those with reversed end–diastolic flow have more poorly vascularized terminal villi, villous stromal hemorrhage, 'hemorrhagic endovasculitis' and abnormally thin-walled fetal stem vessels[25]. In pregnancies with absent end–diastolic frequencies in the Doppler waveform from the umbilical arteries, the capillary loops in placental terminal villi are decreased in number, they are longer and they have fewer branches than in normal pregnancies[27]. The reduced number and maldevelopment of peripheral villi result in a marked impairment of oxygen extraction from the intervillous space. In contrast, placentas from growth-restricted fetuses with positive end–diastolic frequencies have a normal pattern of stem artery development, increased capillary angiogenesis and development of terminal villi, as signs of an adaptative mechanism[28].

Clinical studies of umbilical arterial flow velocity waveforms in intrauterine growth restriction have reported progressive increase in impedance to flow until absence and, in extreme cases, reversal of end–diastolic frequencies (Figure 2)[28–32]. The latter represents the extreme end of the spectrum and this finding is associated with a high perinatal mortality, as well as an increased incidence of lethal fetal structural and chromosomal defects[33,34].

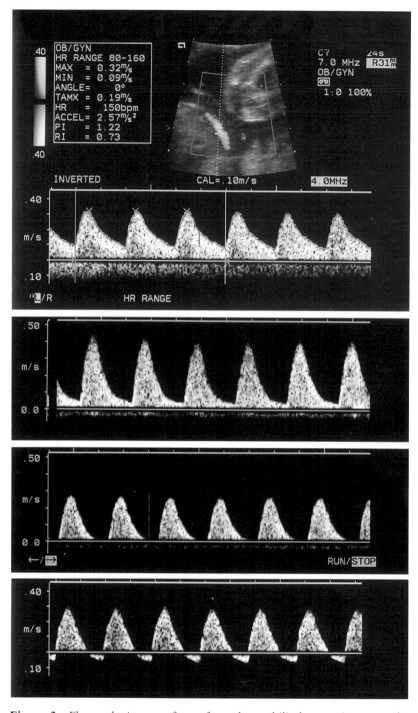

Figure 2 Flow velocity waveforms from the umbilical artery in a growth-restricted fetus demonstrating progressive deterioration from normal waveform (top) to low but positive diastolic flow, absent and finally reversed end–diastolic flow (bottom)

Nicolaides *et al.* measured blood gases in umbilical cord blood samples obtained by cordocentesis in 39 growth-restricted fetuses[12]. End-diastolic frequencies were absent in 22 cases; 80% of these fetuses were found to be hypoxemic and 46% also acidemic. In contrast, only 12% of the fetuses with positive end-diastolic frequencies were hypoxemic and none was acidemic.

In a multicenter study involving high-risk pregnancies, the patients were subdivided into three groups depending on the flow velocity waveforms in the umbilical artery (positive end-diastolic frequencies, $n = 214$; absent end-diastolic frequencies, $n = 178$); and reversed end-diastolic frequencies, $n = 67$)[35]. The overall perinatal mortality rate was 28% and the relative risk was 1.0 for patients with present frequencies, 4.0 for those with absent frequencies and 10.6 for those with reversed frequencies. Significantly more neonates in the groups with absent or reversed frequencies needed admittance to the neonatal intensive care unit and they had a higher risk of cerebral hemorrhage, anemia or hypoglycemia[35]. In addition to increased fetal and neonatal mortality, gowth restriction with absent or reversed end-diastolic frequencies in the umbilical artery is associated with increased incidence of long-term permanent neurological damage[36].

A review of 12 randomized, controlled trials of Doppler ultrasonography of the umbilical artery in high-risk pregnancies reported that, in the Doppler group, there was a significant reduction in the number of antenatal admissions (44%, 95% confidence interval (CI) 28–57%), induction of labor (20%, 95% CI 10–28%), and Cesarean section for fetal distress (52%, 95% CI 24–69%)[37]. Furthermore, the clinical action guided by Doppler ultrasonography reduced the odds of perinatal death by 38% (95% CI 15–55%). Post hoc analyses revealed a statistically significant reduction in elective delivery, intrapartum fetal distress, and hypoxic encephalopathy in the Doppler group. It was concluded that there is now compelling evidence that women with high-risk pregnancies, including pre-eclampsia and suspected intrauterine growth restriction, should be offered Doppler ultrasonographic study of umbilical artery waveforms[37].

In terms of monitoring growth-restricted pregnancies, abnormal waveforms in the umbilical artery are an early sign of fetal impairment. For example, Bekedam *et al.* followed up growth-restricted fetuses longitudinally and reported that abnormalities in the umbilical artery preceded the occurrence of cardiotocographic signs of fetal hypoxemia in more than 90% of cases[38]. The median time interval between absence of end-diastolic frequencies and the onset of late decelerations was 12 days (range 0–49 days).

Fetal arterial blood flow redistribution

In fetal hypoxemia, there is an increase in the blood supply to the brain, myocardium and the adrenal glands and reduction in the perfusion of the kidneys, gastrointestinal tract and the lower extremities (Figures 3 and 4, Table 1)[39–66]. Although knowledge of the factors governing circulatory readjustments and their mechanism of action is

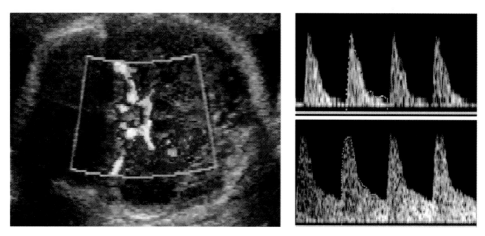

Figure 3 Color Doppler examination of the circle of Willis (left). Flow velocity waveforms from the middle cerebral artery in a normal fetus with low diastolic velocities (right, top) and in a growth-restricted fetus with high diastolic velocities (right, bottom)

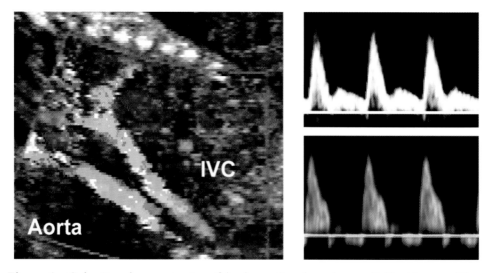

Figure 4 Color Doppler examination of the descending thoracic aorta (left) with normal flow velocity waveforms showing positive flow velocities during diastole (right, top) and in a growth-restricted fetus with reversed end–diastolic velocities (right, bottom)

Table 1 Hemodynamic changes occurring in fetal arterial vessels during hypoxemia and acidemia induced by uteroplacental insufficiency

Vessel	Impedance to flow
Descending aorta	increased
Renal artery	increased
Femoral artery	increased
Peripheral pulmonary artery	increased
Mesenteric arteries	increased
Cerebral arteries	decreased
Adrenal artery	decreased
Splenic artery	decreased
Coronary arteries	decreased

incomplete, it appears that partial pressures of oxygen and carbon dioxide play a role, presumably through their action on chemoreceptors. This mechanism allows preferential delivery of nutrients and oxygen to vital organs, thereby compensating for diminished placental resources. However, compensation through cerebral vasodilatation is limited and a plateau corresponding to a nadir of pulsatility index (PI) in cerebral vessels is reached at least 2 weeks before the development of the fetus is jeopardized. Consequently, arterial vessels are unsuitable for longitudinal monitoring of growth-restricted fetuses. Cardiac and venous velocity waveforms give more information regarding fetal well-being or compromise.

Arduini *et al.* examined growth-restricted fetuses longitudinally and described a curvilinear relationship between impedance in cerebral vessels and the state of fetal oxygenation; the progressive fall in impedance reached a nadir 2 weeks before the onset of late fetal heart rate decelerations[55]. This suggests that the maximum degree of vascular adaptation to hypoxemia precedes the critical degree of impairment of fetal oxygenation. Similarly, Potts *et al.* described a curvilinear relationship between cerebral vascular response and hypercapnia[56]. Vyas *et al.* reported that, concomitant to severe oxygen deficit, there was a sudden rise in middle cerebral artery PI; they suggested that vascular dilatation may be suppressed by the development of cerebral edema[53]. An alternative explanation may be that, in severe hypoxemia, an increase in PI may be the consequence of alterations in flow due to reduced cardiac contractility and to a fall in absolute cardiac output. Moreover, in fetal sheep, chronic hypoxemia was found to alter cerebral vascular contractility through changes in vascular smooth muscle and endothelial cells, with the net result of a relative decrease in cerebral blood flow[57].

Fetal arterial Doppler studies are useful in the differential diagnosis of small-for-gestation fetuses. In the hypoxemic group, due to impaired placental perfusion, the PI in the umbilical artery is increased and, in the fetal middle cerebral artery, the PI is decreased; consequently, the ratio in PI between the umbilical artery and middle cerebral artery (UA/MCA) is increased[58–61]. Bahado-Singh et al. reported that an abnormally low cerebroplacental ratio is associated with increased perinatal morbidity and mortality and that the ratio improves the prediction of perinatal outcome compared with umbilical artery PI alone[65]. However, the cerebroplacental ratio did not appear to correlate significantly with outcome after 34 weeks. In third-trimester fetuses, the ratio in PI between the fetal descending thoracic aorta and the middle cerebral artery may be more useful[66].

There is no evidence that the use of other peripheral arterial fetal vessels, such as renal artery[51], splenic artery[64] or peripheral pulmonary arteries[63] provides any advantage in the identification of intrauterine growth-restricted fetuses.

Fetal cardiac Doppler

Cardiac flow is greatly influenced by the modifications of arterial impedance to flow. Cerebral vasodilatation produces a decrease in left ventricle afterload, whereas increased placental and systemic resistance produce increased right ventricle afterload. Hypoxemia may also impair cardiac contractility directly, while changes in blood viscosity due to polycythemia may alter preload[5]. Consequently, growth-restricted fetuses show, at the level of the atrioventricular valves, impaired ventricular filling (lower ratio of early passive to late active ventricular filling phase – E/A ratio)[67], lower peak velocities in the aorta and pulmonary arteries[68], increased aortic and decreased pulmonary time to peak velocity[69] and a relative increase of left cardiac output associated with decreased right cardiac output[70]. These hemodynamic intracardiac changes are compatible with a preferential shift of cardiac output in favor of the left ventricle, leading to improved cerebral perfusion. Thus, in the first stages of the disease, the supply of substrates and oxygen can be maintained at near normal levels despite any absolute reduction of placental transfer[71].

Longitudinal studies of deteriorating growth-restricted fetuses have shown that peak velocity and cardiac output gradually decline, suggesting a progressive worsening in cardiac function[71]. Similarly, there is a symmetrical decrease in ventricular ejection force at the level of both ventricles, despite the dramatically different hemodynamic conditions present in the vascular district of ejection of the two ventricles (i.e. reduced cerebral resistances for the left ventricle and increased splachnic and placental resistance for the right ventricle)[72]. This supports a pivotal role of the intrinsic myocardial function in the compensatory mechanism of the growth-restricted fetus following the establishment of the brain-sparing effect. Ventricular ejection force dramatically decreases in a short time interval (about 1 week), showing an impairment of ventricular force close to fetal distress. As a consequence, cardiac filling also is impaired.

Fetal venous Doppler

Animal studies have shown that, in severe hypoxemia, there is redistribution in the umbilical venous blood towards the ductus venosus at the expense of hepatic blood flow. Consequently, the proportion of umbilical venous blood contributing to the fetal cardiac output is increased. There is a doubling of umbilical venous-derived oxygen delivery to the myocardium and an increase in oxygen delivery to the fetal brain[73,74]. *In vitro* perfusion studies have shown that, at reduced umbilical venous pressures, a proportionally greater fraction of umbilical venous flow is directed through the ductus venosus in comparison to blood flow through the liver[75]. The same is true during perfusion with blood of high hematocrit. Mechanical forces seem to play a key role in the regulation of umbilical venous flow distribution between the liver and the ductus venosus. Under unfavorable conditions, the ductus venosus seems to ensure blood flow directly to the fetal heart and, in extreme conditions, umbilical blood may pass exclusively through the ductus venosus. This may lead to an impaired perfusion of the liver with potential impact on its metabolic properties. Blood flow measurements with chronically implanted electromagnetic flow transducers in fetal sheep have shown an increase of the amplitude of vena caval pulsations during hypoxemia and increased afterload[76]. Flow waveforms show an increase in peak systolic forward flow, and during atrial contraction retrograde flow occurs. In contrast, reductions in afterload are associated with an increase in peak diastolic forward flow, indicating that fetal systemic vascular resistance has a major influence on venous return and filling patterns of the right heart. Increased placental resistance and peripheral vasoconstriction, as seen in fetal arterial redistribution, cause an increase in right ventricular afterload, and thus ventricular end-diastolic pressure increases. This may result in highly pulsatile venous blood flow waveforms and umbilical venous pulsations due to transmission of atrial pressure waves through the ductus venosus[77].

Studies in growth-restricted human fetuses have demonstrated that, in the inferior vena cava, an increase of reverse flow during atrial contraction occurs with progressive fetal deterioration, suggesting a higher pressure gradient in the right atrium (Figure 5)[78,79]. The next step of the disease is the extension of the abnormal reversal of blood velocities in the inferior vena cava to the ductus venosus, inducing an increase of the S/A ratio, mainly due to a reduction of the A component of the velocity waveforms (Figure 6). Finally, the high venous pressure induces a reduction of velocity at

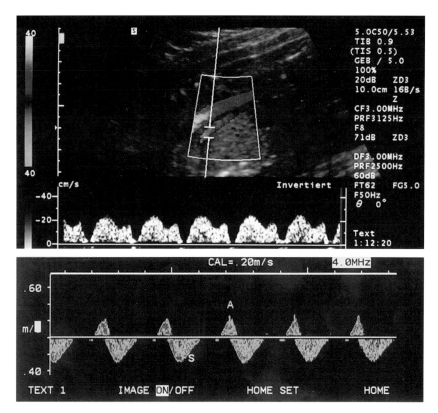

Figure 5 Color Doppler examination of the inferior vena cava with normal flow velocity waveforms (top). Abnormal waveform with increase in reversed flow during atrial contraction in a growth-restricted fetus (bottom)

end-diastole in the umbilical vein, causing typical end-diastolic pulsations (Figure 7)[80]. The development of these pulsations is close to the onset of abnormal fetal heart rate patterns and is frequently associated with acidemia and fetal endocrine changes[81,82]. At this stage, coronary blood flow may be visualized with higher velocity than in normally grown third-trimester fetuses and, if fetuses are not delivered, intrauterine death may occur within a few days[83]. In a study of 37 fetuses with absent end-diastolic frequencies in the umbilical artery, the main factors determining the length of the interval between the first occurrence of absent end-diastolic frequencies were gestational age (the lower the gestation, the longer was the interval), pre-eclampsia (shorter interval) and the presence of pulsations in the umbilical vein; the neonatal mortality in this group with pulsatile venous flow was 63%, compared to 19% in fetuses without pulsations[84].

Fetal venous Doppler studies are useful in monitoring the growth-restricted redistributing fetus. Normal venous flow suggests continuing fetal compensation, whereas abnormal flow indicates the breakdown of hemodynamic compensatory

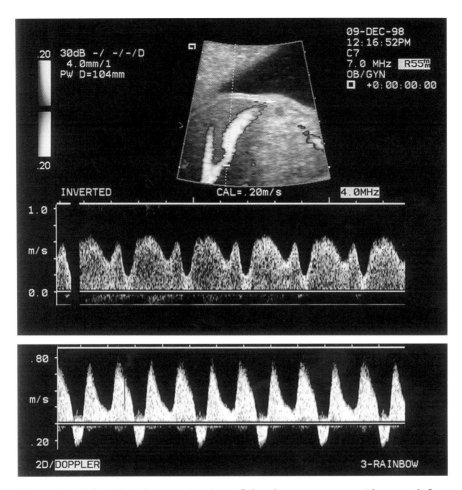

Figure 6 Color Doppler examination of the ductus venosus with normal flow velocity waveforms (top). Abnormal waveform with reversal of flow during atrial contraction and markedly increased pulsatility in a growth-restricted fetus (bottom)

mechanisms[79]. Hecher *et al.* compared fetal venous and arterial blood flow with biophysical assessment in 108 high-risk pregnancies after 23 weeks of gestation[85]. The results of this study suggest that venous Doppler findings in the late third-trimester fetus may not be as reliable as during the late second and early third trimesters. However, the most interesting results were found in a group of 41 fetuses displaying arterial blood flow redistribution. There were no significant differences in arterial PI values between fetuses with normal and abnormal biophysical assessment parameters (except for the aorta and abnormal fetal heart rate trace), whereas venous pulsatility was significantly increased in compromised fetuses compared to the non-compromised group.

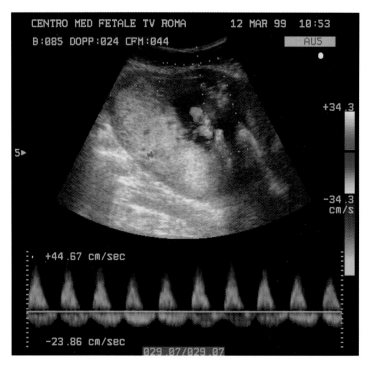

Figure 7 Pulsatile flow in the umbilical vein of a severely compromised growth-restricted fetus

Fetal hypoxemia is associated with a reduction in umbilical venous blood flow, but, despite this decrease, a normal peak velocity in the ductus venosus is maintained[86]. In the growth-restricted fetus, the percentage of umbilical venous blood passing through the ductus venosus is increased from about 40% (in normal fetuses) to about 60%[87]. Therefore, there is a redistribution in venous blood flow in favor of the ductus venosus at the expense of hepatic blood flow. Unlike peak velocity during ventricular systole, there were reduced or even reversed flow velocities during atrial contraction. One may speculate that increased end-diastolic right ventricular pressure would not influence ductus venosus blood flow velocities during atrial contraction, as flow is preferentially directed through the foramen ovale to the left atrium. However, the foramen ovale is closed during atrial contraction and blood flow velocity through the foramen ovale decreases to zero.

Alterations of venous flow velocity waveforms are in a closer temporal relationship to intrauterine fetal jeopardy, compared to changes in arterial flow, which may occur quite early during the course of impaired placental function. The degree of fetal acidemia can be estimated from Doppler measurements of pulsatility in both the arterial system and the ductus venosus. This was shown in a cross-sectional study of 23 severely growth-retstricted fetuses, examining the relationship between Doppler measurements and umbilical venous blood gases obtained at cordocentesis[88]. With moderate acidemia (pH between –2 and –4 standard deviations from the normal mean for gestational age), almost all fetuses had a middle cerebral artery PI below two standard deviations, whereas there was a wide scatter of individual results for the ductus venosus, with the majority of measurements being still within the reference ranges. With increasing severity of hypoxemia and acidemia, ductus venosus PIs increased and, in the most severe cases, velocities with atrial contraction were reduced to zero or even became negative. In a study investigating the association of arterial and venous Doppler findings with adverse perinatal outcome in severe fetal growth restriction, abnormal Doppler velocimetry of the ductus venosus was the only significant parameter associated with perinatal death and low 5-min Apgar scores[89].

There are two possible mechanisms for abnormal venous blood flow waveforms: increasing right ventricular afterload and myocardial failure. As long as the fetus is able to compensate for a reduced placental supply by arterial redistribution, there is preferential myocardial oxygenation, which delays development of right heart failure, despite an increasing afterload. Therefore, fetal Doppler measurements show high placental resistance and arterial redistribution in the presence of normal venous waveforms. At this stage, the majority of fetuses have normal, reactive heart rate traces and biophysical profiles. Progressive changes in the venous circulation may indicate failure of the compensatory mechanism and herald the development of right heart failure due to myocardial hypoxia. Another interesting aspect has been raised by a study examining fetal central venous pressure. The pressure waveform from the inferior vena cava was recorded by following the movement of the vessel wall and thereby recording changes in the vessel lumen diameter[90]. There were two groups of abnormal waveforms: one with a high pulsatile pattern and the other with a shallow and low pulsatile pattern. Both groups had significantly worse clinical outcomes compared to the normal waveform group. However, fetuses in the low pulsatile group were the most severely compromised, all of them showing an abnormal heart rate pattern. It was postulated that impaired contractility and reduced ventricular output, with a concomitantly reduced ventricular filling, were responsible for this waveform pattern.

Timing of delivery

In the management of the very preterm (before 33 weeks of gestation) growth-restricted fetus, there is uncertainty as to whether iatrogenic delivery should be undertaken before the development of signs of severe hypoxemia, with a consequent risk of prematurity-related neonatal complications, or whether delivery should be delayed, but with the risks of prolonged exposure to hypoxia and malnutrition imposed by a hostile intrauterine environment. A growth-restricted fetus leading an ascetic existence from chronic starvation during the late second or early third trimester is capable of tolerating chronic hypoxemia without damage for much longer than a well-nourished late third-trimester fetus with a high energy consumption.

Postnatal follow-up studies, at the age of 7 years, have reported that growth-restricted fetuses with abnormal aortic velocity waveforms had minor neurological dysfunction and impaired intellectual outcome[91,92]. If these findings are confirmed in prospective studies with adequate controls for confounding variables, such as degrees of prematurity, smallness, and management, it may be advisable to deliver growth-restricted fetuses before these blood flow alterations occur. On the other hand, fetuses showing the brain-sparing effect did not have an increased risk for moderate or severe neurological handicap at the age of 2 years[93]. It will always be a challenge to weigh the risks and benefits of early interventions against each other and it is a dynamic process, in which advancements in both fetal and neonatal medicine are of crucial importance for the counselling of parents and the management of these pregnancies.

In the growth-restricted hypoxemic fetus, redistribution of well-oxygenated blood to vital organs, such as the brain, heart and adrenals, represents a compensatory mechanism to prevent fetal damage. When the reserve capacities of the circulatory redistribution reach their limits, fetal deterioration may occur rapidly. In clinical practice, it is necessary to carry out serial Doppler investigations to estimate the duration of fetal blood flow redistribution. The onset of abnormal venous Doppler results indicates deterioration in the fetal condition and iatrogenic delivery should be considered.

In the sequence of deterioration of the condition of the growth-restricted fetus, the first pathological finding is increased impedance to flow in the umbilical artery. This is followed by evidence of arterial redistribution in the fetal circulation and, subsequently, the development of pathological fetal heart rate patterns. On average, the time interval between the onset of abnormal umbilical arterial Doppler results and the onset of late fetal heart rate decelerations is about 2 weeks, but this interval differs considerably among fetuses and is shorter in late than early pregnancy and in the presence of hypertensive disease[31,38,84,94,95]. Increased impedance to flow in the umbilical artery is usually associated with evidence of arterial redistribution in the fetal circulation; this is best monitored by examining the PI in the middle cerebral artery, which is decreased. Late fetal heart rate decelerations are preceded by approximately 2 weeks with Doppler evidence of a nadir in the brain-sparing effect and by a few days with an abrupt increase in impedance in the umbilical arteries[55]. In the first stages of the disease, there is a preferential shift of cardiac output in favor of the left ventricle, leading to improved cerebral perfusion[71], but, with deterioration in the fetal condition, there are a decline in cardiac output and progressive worsening in cardiac function[71]. Normal venous flow suggests continuing fetal compensation, whereas abnormal flow indicates the breakdown of hemodynamic compensatory mechanisms[79]. An abrupt increase in pulsatility of ductus venosus waveforms with loss of forward flow velocity during atrial contraction precede the onset of pathological fetal heart rate patterns and decreased short-term variation. However, the interval may be as short as a few hours in late gestation and in patients with pre-eclampsia; in contrast, during the second trimester, severely abnormal venous waveforms can be present for several days before intrauterine death.

REFERENCES

1. Soothill PW, Nicolaides KH, Rodeck CH, Campbell S. Effect of gestational age on fetal and intervillous blood gas and acid–base values in human pregnancy. *Fetal Ther* 1986;1:168–75

2. Nicolaides KH, Economides DL, Soothill PW. Blood gases and pH and lactate in appropriate and small for gestational age fetuses. *Am J Obstet Gynecol* 1989;161:996–1001

3. Battaglia FC, Meschia G. *An Introduction to Fetal Physiology.* London: Academic Press, 1986:154–67

4. Burd LI, Jones MD, Simmons MA. Placental production and fetal utilisation of lactate and pyruvate. *Nature (London)* 1975;254:210–1

5. Soothill PW, Nicolaides KH, Campbell S. Prenatal asphyxia, hyperlacticaemia, hypoglycaemia and erythroblastosis in growth retarded fetuses. *Br Med J* 1987;294:1051–3

6. Economides DL, Nicolaides KH. Blood glucose and oxygen tension levels in small for gestational age fetuses. *Am J Obstet Gynecol* 1989;160:385–9

7. Economides DL, Proudler A, Nicolaides KH. Plasma insulin in appropriate and small for gestational age fetuses. *Am J Obstet Gynecol* 1989;160:1091–4

8. Economides DL, Nicolaides KH, Gahl W, Bernardini I, Evans M. Plasma amino acids in appropriate and small for gestational age fetuses. *Am J Obstet Gynecol* 1989;161:1219–27

9. Economides DL, Crook D, Nicolaides KH. Hypertriglyceridemia and hypoxemia in small for gestational age fetuses. *Am J Obstet Gynecol* 1990;162:382–6

10. Thorpe-Beeston JG, Nicolaides KH, Snijders RJM, Felton CV, McGregor AM. Thyroid function in small for gestational age fetuses. *Obstet Gynecol* 1991;77:701–6

11. Soothill PW, Nicolaides KH, Bilardo CM, Hackett G, Campbell S. Utero-placental blood flow velocity resistance index and venous pO_2, pCO_2, pH, lactate and erythroblast count in growth retarded fetuses. *Fetal Ther* 1986;l:l76–9

12. Nicolaides KH, Bilardo CM, Soothill PW, Campbell S. Absence of end diastolic frequencies in the umbilical artery: a sign of fetal hypoxia and acidosis. *Br Med J* 1988;297:1026–7

13. Brosens I, Robertson WB, Dixon HG. The role of the spiral arteries in the pathogenesis of pre-eclampsia. *Obstet Gynecol Annu* 1972;1:177–91

14. Giles WB, Trudinger BJ, Baird PJ. Fetal umbilical artery flow velocity waveforms and placental resistance: pathological correlation. *Br J Obstet Gynaecol* 1985;92:31–8

15. Peeters LL, Sheldon RE, Jones MD, Makowsky EL, Meschia G. Blood flow to fetal organs as a function of arterial oxygen content. *Am J Obstet Gynecol* 1979;135:637–46

16. Robertson WB, Brosens I, Dixon HG. The pathological response of the vessels of the placental bed to hypertensive pregnancy. *J Pathol Bacteriol* 1967;93:581–92

17. Sheppard BL, Bonnar J. An ultrastructural study of utero-placental spiral arteries in hypertensive and normotensive pregnancy and fetal growth retardation. *Br J Obstet Gynaecol* 1981;88:695–705

18. Brosens IA. Morphological changes in the utero-placental bed in pregnancy hypertension. *Clin Obstet Gynecol* 1977;4:573–93

19. Khong TY, De Wolf F, Robertson WB, Brosens I. Inadequate maternal vascular response to placentation in pregnancies complicated by pre-eclampsia and by small-for-gestational age infants. *Br J Obstet Gynaecol* 1986;93:1049–59

20. Campbell S, Griffin DR, Pearce JM, Diaz-Recasens J, Cohen-Overbeek T, Wilson K, Teague MJ. New Doppler technique for assessing uteroplacental blood flow. *Lancet* 1983;26:675–7

21. Trudinger BJ, Giles WB, Cook CM. Uteroplacental blood flow velocity-time waveforms in normal and complicated pregnancy. *Br J Obstet Gynaecol* 1985;92:39–45

22. Campbell S, Pearce JM, Hackett G, Cohen-Overbeek T, Hernandez C. Qualitative assessment of uteroplacental blood flow: an early screening test for high risk pregnancies. *Obstet Gynecol* 1986;68: 649–53

23. Fleisher A, Schulman H, Farmakides G, Bracero L, Rochelson B, Koenigsberg M. Uterine artery Doppler velocimetry in pregnant women with hypertension. *Am J Obstet Gynecol* 1986;154:806–13

24. Karsdorp VH, Dirks BK, van der Linden JC, van Vugt JM, Baak JP, van Geijn HP. Placenta morphology and absent or reversed end diastolic flow velocities in the umbilical artery: a clinical and morphometrical study. *Placenta* 1996;17:393–9

25. Salafia CM, Pezzullo JC, Minior VK, Divon MY. Placental pathology of absent and reversed end-diastolic flow in growth-restricted fetuses. *Obstet Gynecol* 1997;90:830–6

26. Schulman H, Fleisher A, Stern W, Farmakides G, Jagani N, Blattner P. Umbilical velocity wave ratios in human pregnancy. *Am J Obstet Gynecol* 1984;148:985–90

27. Krebs C, Macara LM, Leiser R, Bowman AW, Greer IA, Kingdom JCP. Intrauterine growth restriction with absent end-diastolic flow velocity in the umbilical artery is associated with mal-development of the placental terminal villous tree. *Am J Obstet Gynecol* 1996;175:1534–42

28. Todros T, Sciarrone A, Piccoli E, Guiot C, Kaufmann P, Kingdom J. Umbilical Doppler waveforms and placental villous angiogenesis in pregnancies complicated by fetal growth restriction. *Obstet Gynecol* 1999;93:499–503

29. Erskine RL, Ritchie JW. Umbilical artery blood flow characteristics in normal and growth retarded fetuses. *Br J Obstet Gynaecol* 1985;92:605–10

30. Trudinger BJ, Giles WB, Cook CM, Bombardieri J, Collins L. Fetal umbilical artery flow velocity waveforms and placental resistance: clinical significance. *Br J Obstet Gynaecol* 1985;92:23–30

31. Reuwer PJ, Sijmons EA, Rietman GW, van Tiel MW, Bruinse HW. Intrauterine growth retardation: prediction of perinatal distress by Doppler ultrasound. *Lancet* 1987;22:415–18

32. Rochelson B, Shulman H, Farmakides G, Bracero L, Ducey J, Fleisher A, Penny B, Winter D. The significance of absent end-diastolic velocity in umbilical artery velocity waveforms. *Am J Obstet Gynecol* 1987;156:1213–38

33. Mandruzzato GP, Bogatti P, Fischer L, Gigli C. The clinical significance of absent or reverse end-diastolic flow in the fetal aorta and umbilical artery. *Ultrasound Obstet Gynecol* 1991;1:192–6

34. Brar HS, Platt LD. Reverse end-diastolic flow velocity on umbilical artery velocimetry in high risk pregnancies: an ominous finding with adverse pregnancy outcome. *Am J Obstet Gynecol* 1988;159: 559–61

35. Karsdorp VH, van Vugt JM, van Geijn HP, Kostense PJ, Arduini D, Montenegro N, Todros T. Clinical significance of absent or reversed end diastolic velocity waveforms in umbilical artery. *Lancet* 1994;344:1664–8

36. Valcamonico A, Danti L, Frusca T, Soregaroli M, Zucca S, Abrami F, Tiberti A. Absent end-diastolic velocity in umbilical artery: risk of neonatal morbidity and brain damage. *Am J Obstet Gynecol* 1994;170:796–801

37. Alfirevic Z, Neilson JP. Doppler ultrasonography in high-risk pregnancies: systematic review with meta-analysis. *Am J Obstet Gynecol* 1995;172:1379–87

38. Bekedam DJ, Visser GHA, van der Zee AGJ, Snijders RJM, Poelmann-Weesjes G. Abnormal velocity waveforms of the umbilical artery in growth-retarded fetuses: relationship to antepartum late heart rate decelerations and outcome. *Early Hum Dev* 1990;24:79–89

39. Soothill PW, Nicolaides KH, Bilardo KM, Campbell S. The relationship of fetal hypoxia in growth retardation to the mean blood velocity in the fetal aorta. *Lancet* 1986;2:1118–20

40. Wladimiroff JW, Tonge HM, Stewart PA. Doppler ultrasound assessment of cerebral blood flow in the human fetus. *Br J Obstet Gynaecol* 1986;93:471–5

41. Tonge HM, Wladimiroff JW, Noordam MJ, van Kooten C. Blood flow velocity waveforms in the descending fetal aorta: comparison between normal and growth retarded pregnancies. *Obstet Gynecol* 1986;67:851–5

42. van Eyck J, Wladimiroff JW, Noordam MJ, Tonge HM, Prechtl HFR. The blood flow velocity waveform in the fetal descending aorta: its relationship to behavioural states in growth retarded fetus at 37–38 weeks of gestation. *Early Hum Dev* 1986;14:99–107

43. Wladimiroff JW, van Wijngaard JAGW, Degani S, Noordam MJ, van Eijck J, Tonge HM. Cerebral and umbilical arterial blood flow velocity waveforms in normal and growth retarded pregnancies. *Obstet Gynecol* 1987;69:705–9

44. Laurin J, Lingman G, Marsal K, Persson PH. Fetal blood flow in pregnancies complicated by intrauterine growth retardation. *Obstet Gynecol* 1987;69:895–902

45. Laurin J, Marsal K, Persson P, Lingman H. Ultrasound measurements of fetal blood flow in predicting fetal outcome. *Br J Obstet Gynaecol* 1987;94:940–8

46. Arduini D, Rizzo D, Romanini C, Mancuso S. Fetal blood flow velocity waveforms as predictors of growth retardation. *Obstet Gynecol* 1987;70:7–10

47. van Eyck J, Wladimiroff JW, van den Wijngaard JAGW, Noordam MJ, Prechtl HFR. The blood flow velocity waveform in the internal carotid artery: its relationship to behavioural states in growth retarded fetus at 37–38 weeks of gestation. *Br J Obstet Gynaecol* 1987;94:736–41

48. Arabin B, Bergmann PL, Saling E. Simultaneous assessment of blood flow velocity waveforms in uteroplacental vessels, umbilical artery, fetal aorta and common carotid artery. *Fetal Ther* 1987;2: 17–26

49. Hackett G, Campbell S, Gamsu H, Cohen-Overbeek T, Pearce JMF. Doppler studies in the growth retarded fetus and prediction of neonatal necrotising enterocolitis, haemorrhage, and neonatal morbidity. *Br Med J* 1987;294:13–16

50. Bilardo CM, Campbell S, Nicolaides KH. Mean blood velocities and impedance in the fetal descending thoracic aorta and common carotid artery in normal pregnancy. *Early Hum Dev* 1988; 18:213–21

51. Vyas S, Nicolaides KH, Campbell S. Renal artery flow velocity waveforms in normal and hypoxemic fetuses. *Am J Obstet Gynecol* 1989;161:168–72

52. Bilardo CM, Nicolaides KH, Campbell S. Doppler measurements of fetal and uteroplacental circulations: relationship with umbilical venous blood gases measured at cordocentesis. *Am J Obstet Gynecol* 1990;162:115–20

53. Vyas S, Nicolaides KH, Bower S, Campbell S. Middle cerebral artery flow velocity waveforms in fetal hypoxemia. *Br J Obstet Gynaecol* 1990;97:797–803

54. Vyas S, Campbell S, Bower S, Nicolaides KH. Maternal abdominal pressure alters fetal cerebral blood flow. *Br J Obstet Gynaecol* 1990;97:740–2

55. Arduini D, Rizzo G, Romanini C. Changes of pulsatility index from fetal vessels preceding the onset of late decelerations in growth-retarded fetuses. *Obstet Gynecol* 1992;79:605–10

56. Potts P, Connors G, Gillis S, Hunse C, Richardson B. The effect of carbon dioxide on Doppler flow velocity waveforms in the human fetus. *J Dev Physiol* 1992;17:119–23

57. Longo LD, Pearce WJ Fetal and newborn cerebral vascular responses and adaptations to hypoxia. *Semin Perinatol* 1991;15:49–57

58. Arduini D, Rizzo G. Prediction of fetal outcome in small for gestational age fetuses: comparison of Doppler measurements obtained from different fetal vessels. *J Perinat Med* 1992;20:29–38

59. Hecher K, Spernol R, Stettner H, Szalay S. Potential for diagnosing imminent risk to appropriate- and small-for-gestational-age fetuses by Doppler sonographic examination of umbilical and cerebral arterial blood flow. *Ultrasound Obstet Gynecol* 1992;2:266–71

60. Gramellini D, Folli MC, Raboni S, Vadora E, Merialdi A. Cerebral–umbilical Doppler ratio as a predictor of adverse perinatal outcome. *Obstet Gynecol* 1992;74:416–20

61. Arias F. Accuracy of the middle-cerebral-to-umbilical-artery resistance index ratios in the prediction of neonatal outcome in patients at high risk for fetal and neonatal complications. *Am J Obstet Gynecol* 1994;171:1541–5

62. Akalin-Sel T, Nicolaides KH, Peacock J, Campbell S. Doppler dynamics and their complex interrelation with fetal oxygen pressure, carbon dioxide pressure, and pH in growth-retarded fetuses. *Obstet Gynecol* 1994;84:439–44

63. Rizzo G, Capponi A, Chaoui R, Taddei F, Arduini D, Romanini C. Blood flow velocity waveforms from peripheral pulmonary arteries in normally grown and growth-retarded fetuses. *Ultrasound Obstet Gynecol* 1996;8:87–92

64. Capponi A, Rizzo G, Arduini D, Romanini C. Splenic artery velocity waveforms in small for gestational age fetuses: relationship with pH and blood gases measured in umbilical blood at cordocentesis. *Am J Obstet Gynecol* 1997;176:300–7

65. Bahado-Singh RO, Kovanci E, Jeffres A, Oz U, Deren O, Copel J, Mari G. The Doppler cerebroplacental ratio and perinatal outcome in intrauterine growth restriction. *Am J Obstet Gynecol* 1999;180:750–6

66. Harrington K, Thompson MO, Carpenter RG, Nguyen M, Campbell S. In third trimester fetuses the ratio in pulsatility index between the fetal descending thoracic aorta and the middle cerebral artery may be more useful. Doppler fetal circulation in pregnancies complicated by pre-eclampsia

or delivery of a small for gestational age baby. 2. Longitudinal analysis. *Br J Obstet Gynaecol* 1999; 106:453–66

67. Rizzo G, Arduini D, Romanini C, Mancuso S. Doppler echocardiographic assessment of atrioventricular velocity waveforms in normal and small for gestational age fetuses. *Br J Obstet Gynaecol* 1988;95:65–9

68. Groenenberg IA, Baerts W, Hop WC, Wladimiroff JW. Relationship between fetal cardiac and extra-cardiac Doppler flow velocity waveforms and neonatal outcome in intrauterine growth retardation. *Early Hum Dev* 1991;26:185–92

69. Rizzo G, Arduini D, Romanini C, Mancuso S. Doppler echocardiographic evaluation of time to peak velocity in the aorta and pulmonary artery of small for gestational age fetuses. *Br J Obstet Gynaecol* 1990;97:603–7

70. Al-Ghazaii W, Chita SK, Chapman MG, Allan LD. Evidence of redistribution of cardiac output in asymmetrical growth retardation. *Br J Obstet Gynaecol* 1989;96:697–70

71. Rizzo G, Arduini D. Fetal cardiac function in intrauterine growth retardation. *Am J Obstet Gynecol* 1991;165:876–82

72. Rizzo G, Capponi A, Rinaldo D, Arduini D, Romanini C. Ventricular ejection force in growth retarded fetuses. *Ultrasound Obstet Gynecol* 1995;5:247–55

73. Reuss ML, Rudolph AM. Distribution and recirculation of umbilical and systemic venous blood flow in fetal lambs during hypoxia. *J Dev Physiol* 1980;2:71–84

74. Tchirikov M, Eisermann K, Rybakowski C, Schröder HJ. Doppler ultrasound evaluation of ductus venosus blood flow during acute hypoxemia in fetal lambs. *Ultrasound Obstet Gynecol* 1998;11: 426–31

75. Kiserud T, Stratford L, Hanson MA. Umbilical flow distribution to the liver and the ductus venosus: an *in vitro* investigation of the fluid dynamic mechanism in the fetal sheep. *Am J Obstet Gynecol* 1997;177:86–90

76. Reuss ML, Rudolph AM, Dae MW. Phasic blood flow patterns in the superior and inferior venae cavae and umbilical vein of fetal sheep. *Am J Obstet Gynecol* 1983;145:70–8

77. Kiserud T, Crowe C, Hanson M. Ductus venosus agenesis prevents transmission of central venous pulsations to the umbilical vein in fetal sheep. *Ultrasound Obstet Gynecol* 1998;11:190–4

78. Rizzo G, Arduini D, Romanini C. Inferior vena cava flow velocity waveforms in appropriate and small for gestational age fetuses. *Am J Obstet Gynecol* 1992;166:1271–80

79. Hecher K, Hackeloer BJ. Cardiotocogram compared to Doppler investigation of the fetal circulation in the premature growth-retarded fetus: longitudinal observations. *Ultrasound Obstet Gynecol* 1997;9:152–61

80. Gudmundusson S, Tulzer G, Huhta JC, Marsal K. Venous Doppler in the fetus with absent end diastolic flow in umbilical artery. *Ultrasound Obstet Gynecol* 1996;7:262–7

81. Rizzo G, Capponi A, Soregaroli M, Arduini D, Romanini C. Umbilical vein pulsations and acid base status at cordocentesis in growth retarded fetuses with absent end diastolic velocity in umbilical artery. *Biol Neonate* 1995;68:163–8

82. Capponi A, Rizzo G, De Angelis C, Arduini D, Romanini C. Atrial natriuretic peptide levels in fetal blood in relation to inferior vena cava velocity waveforms. *Obstet Gynecol* 1997;89:242–7

83. Baschat AA, Gembruch U, Reiss I, Gortner L, Diedrich K. Demonstration of fetal coronary blood flow by Doppler ultrasound in relation to arterial and venous flow velocity waveforms and perinatal outcome. The heart sparing effect. *Ultrasound Obstet Gynecol* 1997;9:162–72

84. Arduini D, Rizzo G, Romanini C. The development of abnormal heart rate patterns after absent end-diastolic velocity in umbilical artery: analysis of risk factors. *Am J Obstet Gynecol* 1993;168: 43–50

85. Hecher K, Campbell S, Doyle P, Harrington K, Nicolaides KH. Assessment of fetal compromise by Doppler ultrasound investigation of the fetal circulation. Arterial, intracardiac, and venous blood flow velocity studies. *Circulation* 1995;91:129–38

86. Kiserud T, Eik-Nes SH, Blaas HG, Hellevik LR, Simensen B. Ductus venosus blood velocity and the umbilical circulation in the seriously growth-retarded fetus. *Ultrasound Obstet Gynecol* 1994;4: 109–14

87. Tchirikov M, Rybakowski C, Hüneke B, Schröder HJ. Blood flow through the ductus venosus in singleton and multifetal pregnancies and in fetuses with intrauterine growth retardation. *Am J Obstet Gynecol* 1998;178:943–9

88. Hecher K, Snijders R, Campbell S, Nicolaides KH. Fetal venous, intracardiac, and arterial blood flow measurements in intrauterine growth retardation: relationship with fetal blood gases. *Am J Obstet Gynecol* 1995;173:10–15

89. Ozcan T, Sbracia M, d'Ancona RL, Copel JA, Mari G. Arterial and venous Doppler velocimetry in the severely growth-restricted fetus and association with adverse perinatal outcome. *Ultrasound Obstet Gynecol* 1998;12:39–44

90. Mori A, Trudinger B, Mori R, Reed V, Takeda Y. The fetal central venous pressure waveform in normal pregnancy and in umbilical placental insufficiency. *Am J Obstet Gynecol* 1995;172:51–7

91. Ley D, Laurin J, Bjerre I, Marsal K. Abnormal fetal aortic velocity waveform and minor neurological dysfunction at 7 years of age. *Ultrasound Obstet Gynecol* 1996;8:152–9

92. Ley D, Tideman E, Laurin J, Bjerre I, Marsal K. Abnormal fetal aortic velocity waveform and intellectual function at 7 years of age. *Ultrasound Obstet Gynecol* 1996;8:160–5

93. Chan FY, Pun TC, Lam P, Lam C, Lee CP, Lam YH. Fetal cerebral Doppler studies as a predictor of perinatal outcome and subsequent neurologic handicap. *Obstet Gynecol* 1996;87:981–8

94. Divon MY, Girz BA, Lieblich R, Langer O. Clinical management of the fetus with markedly diminished umbilical artery end-diastolic flow. *Am J Obstet Gynecol* 1989;161:1523–7

95. Arabin B, Siebert M, Jimenez E, Saling E. Obstetrical characteristics of a loss of end-diastolic velocities in the fetal aorta and/or umbilical artery using Doppler ultrasound. *Gynecol Obstet Invest* 1988;25:173–80

5

Screening for placental insufficiency by uterine artery Doppler

INTRODUCTION

Impaired trophoblastic invasion of the maternal spiral arteries is associated with increased risk for subsequent development of intrauterine growth restriction, pre-eclampsia and placental abruption (see Chapter 4). A series of screening studies involving assessment of impedance to flow in the uterine arteries have examined the potential value of Doppler in identifying pregnancies at risk of the complications of impaired placentation (Figures 1–3).

STUDIES IN SELECTED POPULATIONS

Arduini *et al.* examined 60 women who had essential hypertension or renal disease or a previous pregnancy complicated by pregnancy-induced hypertension[1]. They

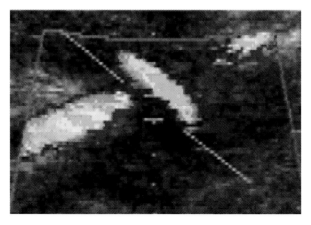

Figure 1   Insonation of the uterine artery at the crossover with the iliac artery

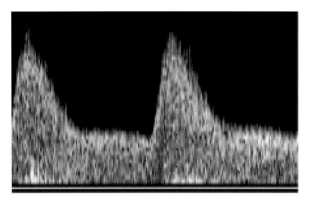

Figure 2 Normal flow velocity waveform from the uterine artery at 24 weeks of gestation

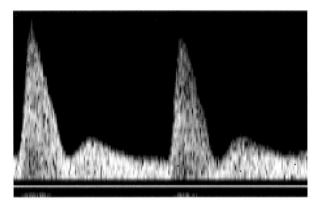

Figure 3 Flow velocity waveform from the uterine artery at 24 weeks of gestation in a pregnancy with impaired placentation; in early diastole there is a notch and in late diastole there is decreased flow

measured impedance to flow in the arcuate arteries at 18–20 weeks of gestation and defined as an abnormal result a resistance index of more than 0.57. They reported that this test identified 64% of pregnancies that subsequently developed pregnancy-induced hypertension (Table 1).

In a similar study, Jacobson et al. examined 91 women who had chronic hypertension, history of pre-eclampsia or fetal loss and a variety of other medical conditions[2]. They measured impedance to flow in the arcuate arteries at 24 weeks of gestation and defined as an abnormal result a resistance index of more than 0.57. Doppler signals could not be obtained in 8% of women and these pregnancies were considered to have abnormal test results. The sensitivity of the test for pregnancy-induced hypertension was 44% (Table 1). This study also examined prediction of intrauterine growth

Table 1 Screening for pregnancy-induced hypertension in high-risk pregnancies by measurement of impedance to flow in the arcuate or uterine arteries

	Arduini et al., 1987[1]	Jacobson et al., 1990[2]	Zimmermann et al., 1997[3]
Gestation at Doppler	18–20 weeks	24 weeks	21–24 weeks
Patients	60	91	172
Prevalence of pre-eclampsia	37%	29%	18%
Sensitivity	64%	44%	56%
Specificity	94%	73%	83%
Positive predictive value	70%	33%	43%
Negative predictive value	80%	81%	89%

restriction (birth weight below the 10th centile for gestation), which was found in 18% of the cases and the sensitivity and positive predictive values were 71% and 33%, respectively.

Zimmermann et al. examined 172 women at high risk for hypertensive disorders of pregnancy or intrauterine growth restriction[3]. They measured impedance to flow in the uterine arteries at 21–24 weeks of gestation and defined an abnormal result by a resistance index of more than 0.68. The prevalence of pre-eclampsia and/or intrauterine growth restriction was 18% and the sensitivity of increased impedance in the prediction of this complication was 56% (Table 1).

STUDIES IN UNSELECTED POPULATIONS

Several studies in unselected populations have examined the value of Doppler assessment of the uteroplacental circulation in the prediction of pre-eclampsia and/or intrauterine growth restriction. The main characteristics and results of the studies are summarized in Tables 2–4. The early studies were limited by the use of continuous wave Doppler, which is a blind investigation. However, recent studies have used color Doppler ultrasound to assess flow in the uterine artery at the point where it crosses the external iliac artery, which is a more reproducible examination. Discrepant results between the studies may be the consequence of differences in Doppler technique for sampling and the definition of abnormal flow velocity waveform, differences in the populations examined (for example, the prevalence of pre-eclampsia varied from as low as 2% to as high as 24%), the gestational age at which women were studied, and different criteria for the diagnosis of pre-eclampsia and intrauterine growth restriction.

Table 2 Characteristics of uteroplacental Doppler screening studies in unselected populations. Under Abnormal result, the values are given as resistance index (RI) equivalent

Author	n	Doppler	Vessel	Abnormal result	Gestational age (weeks)
One-stage screening					
Campbell et al., 1986[4]	126	PW	arcuate arteries	RI > 0.58	16–18
Hanretty et al., 1989[5]	291	CW	arcuate arteries	RI > 0.52	26–30
Bewley et al., 1991[6]	925	CW	uterine and arcuate arteries	mean RI > 95th centile	16–24
Bower et al., 1993[7]	2058	CW	uterine	RI > 95th centile or notch	18–22
Valensise et al., 1993[8]	272	color	uterine	mean RI > 0.58	22
North et al., 1994[9]	457	color	uterine (placental side)	RI > 0.57	19–24
Chan et al., 1995[10]	334	CW	uterine arteries	RI > 90th centile and bilateral notches	20
Irion et al., 1998[11]	1159	color	uterine (placental side)	mean RI > 0.57	26
Kurdi et al., 1998[12]	946	color	uterine arteries	RI > 0.55 and bilateral notches	19–21
Two-stage screening					
Steel et al., 1990[13]	1014	CW/CW	uterine arteries	RI > 0.58	18 and 24
Bower et al., 1993[14]	2437	CW/color	uterine arteries	RI > 95th centile or notches	20 and 24
Harrington et al., 1996[15]	1233	CW/color	uterine	RI > 95th centile or notches	20 and 24
Frusca et al., 1997[16]	419	CW/color	uterine arteries	mean RI > 0.58	20 and 24

PW, Pulsed wave; CW, continuous wave

One-stage screening

Arcuate arteries

Campbell *et al.* examined the arcuate arteries in 126 pregnancies at 16–18 weeks of gestation[4]. Subsequently, 12% of cases developed pre-eclampsia and 14% developed intrauterine growth restriction. The sensitivity of increased impedance (resistance index of more than 0.58) in the prediction of pre-eclampsia was 67% and, for intrauterine growth restriction, it was also 67%; the specificity was about 65% for both. In contrast, Hanretty *et al.* examined the arcuate arteries in 291 pregnancies at 26–30 weeks of gestation and found no difference in pregnancy outcome between those with normal and abnormal Doppler results[5].

Table 3 Results of uteroplacental Doppler screening studies for the prediction of pre-eclampsia (PET) in unselected populations providing data on prevalence, sensitivity, specificity, positive predictive value (PPV) and negative predictive value (NPV)

Author	Outcome measure	Prevalence (%)	Sensitivity (%)	Specificity (%)	PPV (%)	NPV (%)
One-stage screening						
Campbell *et al.*, 1986[4]	PET 1	11.9	67	64	20	93
Hanretty *et al.*, 1989[5]	PET 2	24.1	7	94	26	76
Bewley *et al.*, 1991[6]	PET 3	4.6	24	95	20	96
Bower *et al.*, 1993[7]	PET 4	2.5	75	86	12	99
Valensise *et al.*, 1993[8]	PET 4	3.3	89	93	31	99
North *et al.*, 1994[9]	PET 4	3.3	27	90	8	97
Chan *et al.*, 1995[10]	PET 5	6.9	22	97	36	94
Irion *et al.*, 1998[11]	PET 4	4.0	26	88	7	
Kurdi *et al.*, 1998[12]	PET 3	2.2	62	89	11	99
Two-stage screening						
Steel *et al.*, 1990[13]	PET 4	1.9	63	89	10	99
Bower *et al.*, 1993[14]	PET 4	1.8	78	95	22	99
Harrington *et al.*, 1996[15]	PET 6	3.6	77	94	31	99
Frusca *et al.*, 1997[16]	PET 4	1.9	50	92	11	99

Definitions of hypertensive disease (PET) used by the different studies:

PET 1   Blood pressure rise (systolic > 30 mmHg or diastolic > 15 mmHg) with proteinuria or generalized edema

PET 2   Blood pressure ≥ 140/90 mmHg, requiring further investigation or treatment

PET 3   Blood pressure ≥ 140/90 mmHg and proteinuria (> 150 mg/24 h)

PET 4   Blood pressure ≥ 140/90 mmHg and proteinuria (> 300 mg/24 h)

PET 5   Blood pressure ≥ 140/90 mmHg and proteinuria (> 300 mg/24 h) or non-proteinuric hypertension before 37 weeks

PET 6   Blood pressure rise (systolic > 30 mmHg and diastolic > 25 mmHg) with proteinuria (> 500 mg/24 h)

Table 4 Results of uteroplacental Doppler screening studies for the prediction of intrauterine growth restriction (IUGR) in unselected populations providing data on prevalence, sensitivity, specificity, positive predictive value (PPV) and negative predictive value (NPV)

Author	Outcome measure	Prevalence (%)	Sensitivity (%)	Specificity (%)	PPV (%)	NPV (%)
One-stage screening						
Campbell *et al.*, 1986[4]	IUGR < 10th centile	14.3	67	65	24	92
Hanretty *et al.*, 1989[5]	IUGR < 5th centile	5.5	6	93	5	95
Bewley *et al.*, 1991[6]	IUGR < 5th centile	5.7	19	95	19	95
Bower *et al.*, 1993[7]	IUGR < 5th centile	5.2	46	86	15	97
Valensise *et al.*, 1993[8]	IUGR < 10th centile	7.7	67	95	54	97
North *et al.*, 1994[9]	IUGR < 10th centile	6.6	47	91	27	96
Irion *et al.*, 1998[11]	IUGR < 10th centile	11	29	89	25	
Kurdi *et al.*, 1998[12]	IUGR < 5th centile	6.0	37	89	22	95
Two-stage screening						
Steel *et al.*, 1990[13]	IUGR < 5th centile	7.2	37	90	23	95
Bower *et al.*, 1993[14]	IUGR < 5th centile	4.9	30	95	23	96
Harrington *et al.*, 1996[15]	IUGR < 10th centile	10.6	32	94	38	92
Frusca *et al.*, 1997[16]	IUGR < 10th centile	7.2	43	94	36	96

Uterine and arcuate arteries

Bewley *et al.* calculated the average resistance index from the left and right uterine and arcuate arteries in 925 pregnancies at 16–24 weeks gestation[6]. When the resistance index was greater than the 95th centile, there was a 10-fold increase in risk for a severe adverse outcome, defined by fetal death, placental abruption, intrauterine growth restriction or pre-eclampsia (prevalence 7%, sensitivity 21%, specificity 95%, positive predictive value 25%). However, the sensitivity of the test for pre-eclampsia or intrauterine growth restriction was only 24% and 19%, respectively with a specificity of about 95% for both.

Uterine arteries

Bower *et al.* examined the uterine arteries in 2058 pregnancies at 18–22 weeks[7]. An abnormal result, defined by a resistance index above the 95th centile or the presence of an early diastolic notch in either of the two uterine arteries, was found in 16% of the pregnancies. The sensitivity of the test was 75% for pre-eclampsia and 46% for intrauterine growth restriction, and the specificity was 86% for both. This study highlighted the fact that abnormal Doppler results provide a better prediction of the more severe types of pregnancy complications. Thus, the sensitivity for mild pre-eclampsia was only 29%, but for moderate/severe disease the sensitivity was 82%. Similarly, the sensitivity for birth weight below the 10th centile was 38% and, for birth weight below the 5th centile, it was 46%.

Valensise et al. examined the uterine arteries in 272 primigravidas at 22 weeks of gestation[8]. An abnormal result, defined by increased impedance (mean resistance index of more than 0.58) was found in 9.6% of patients. The sensitivity of the test in predicting pre-eclampsia was 89% and for intrauterine growth restriction it was 67%; the specificities were 93% and 95%, respectively. The sensitivity for predicting non-proteinuric pregnancy-induced hypertension was 50%.

North et al. examined the uterine arteries at 19–24 weeks of gestation in 457 nulliparous women and they found increased impedance (resistance index greater than 0.57 on the placental side) in 11% of cases[9]. The sensitivity of the test for pre-eclampsia was 27%, and for intrauterine growth restriction it was 47%; the respective specificities were 90% and 91%. The test detected women with severe disease requiring delivery before 37 weeks with a sensitivity of 83% and specificity of 88%.

Chan et al. examined the uterine arteries at 20 weeks of gestation in 334 patients considered to be at medium risk for the development of pregnancy-induced hypertension[10]. A screen-positive result, defined by a mean resistance index above the 90th centile and the presence of diastolic notches in both uterine arteries, was found in 4.2% of cases. The sensitivity of the test for pre-eclampsia was 22%, with a specificity of 97% and a positive predictive value of 35.7%.

Irion et al. examined the uterine arteries in 1159 nulliparous women at 26 weeks[11]. Pre-eclampsia, intrauterine growth restriction and preterm delivery occurred in 4%, 11% and 7% of the pregnancies, respectively. At 26 weeks, increased impedance to flow (resistance index greater than 0.57) was present in 13% of cases and the sensitivity of the test was 26% for pre-eclampsia, 29% for growth restriction and 15% for preterm delivery.

Kurdi et al. examined the uterine arteries by color Doppler in 946 unselected women at 19–21 weeks of gestation[12]. In 12.4% of cases, there were bilateral notches and, in this group, the odds ratio for developing pre-eclampsia was 12.8, and, for pre-eclampsia requiring delivery before 37 weeks, it was 52.6. When the uterine artery Doppler studies were normal, the odds ratio for developing pre-eclampsia was 0.11 and, for intrauterine growth restriction (birth weight below the 5th centile for gestation), it was 0.3. In women with bilateral notches and a mean resistance index greater than 0.55, the sensitivities for pre-eclampsia and fetal growth restriction were

62% and 37%, respectively and, for these complications requiring delivery before 37 weeks, the sensitivities were 88% for both. It was concluded that women with normal uterine artery Doppler studies at 20 weeks constitute a group that have a low risk of developing obstetric complications related to uteroplacental insufficiency, whereas women with bilateral notches have an increased risk of the subsequent development of such complications, in particular those requiring delivery before term. Consequently, the results of Doppler studies of the uterine arteries at the time of the routine 20-week anomaly scan may be of use in determining the type and level of antenatal care that is offered to women.

Two-stage screening

Steel *et al.* examined the uterine arteries in 1014 nulliparous women by continuous wave Doppler at 18 weeks of gestation and, in those with increased impedance (resistance index greater than 0.58), the Doppler studies were repeated at 24 weeks[13]. A screen-positive result (increased impedance at 24 weeks) was found in 12% of cases, and the sensitivity of the test for pre-eclampsia was 63% and for intrauterine growth restriction it was 43% (< 5th centile).

Bower *et al.* examined the uterine arteries in 2437 unselected women by continuous wave Doppler at 20 weeks of gestation[14]. In those with increased impedance to flow (resistance index greater than the 95th centile or early diastolic notch in either of the two uterine arteries), the Doppler studies were repeated by color Doppler at 24 weeks. Persistently increased impedance was observed in 5.4% of the patients (compared to 16% at 20 weeks). It was reported that increased impedance provides good prediction of pre-eclampsia (but not of non-proteinuric pregnancy-induced hypertension). Furthermore, in terms of low birth weight, abnormal waveforms provide better prediction of severe (below the 3rd centile) rather than mild (below the 10th centile) intrauterine growth restriction (Table 5).

Harrington *et al.* examined the uterine arteries in 1233 unselected women by continuous wave Doppler at 20 weeks of gestation[15]. In those with increased impedance (resistance index greater than the 95th centile or early diastolic notch in either of the uterine arteries), the Doppler studies were repeated by color Doppler at 24 weeks. Persistently increased impedance was observed in 8.9% of the patients. The sensitivity of the test for pre-eclampsia was 77%, and for intrauterine growth restriction it was 32%. Bilateral notching at 24 weeks was observed in 3.9% of patients; the sensitivity for pre-eclampsia was 55%, and for intrauterine growth restriction it was 22%. The respective sensitivities for those complications leading to delivery before 35 weeks were 81% and 58%.

Table 5 The prediction of complications of pregnancy by increased impedance to flow in the uterine arteries at 24 weeks[14]

Outcome	Prevalence (%)	Sensitivity (%)	Specificity (%)	PPV (%)	NPV (%)
Pregnancy-induced hypertension	6.5	8	94	9	94
Pre-eclampsia	1.8	78	95	22	99
SGA < 3rd centile	3.4	36	95	19	98
SGA < 5th centile	4.9	30	95	23	96
SGA < 10th centile	10.3	23	96	37	92

PPV, positive predictive value; NPV, negative predictive value; SGA, small for gestational age

Frusca *et al.* examined the uterine arteries in 419 nulliparous women by continuous wave Doppler at 20 weeks of gestation[16]. In those with increased mean resistance index (greater than 0.58), the uterine arteries were examined by color Doppler at 24 weeks. Persistently high resistance was observed in 8.6% of the patients. The sensitivity of the test for pre-eclampsia was 50%, and for intrauterine growth restriction it was 43%. In the group with increased impedance at 20 weeks but normal results at 24 weeks, the prevalence of pregnancy complications was not increased compared to those with normal impedance at 20 weeks.

One-stage screening at 23 weeks

Albaiges *et al.* used color Doppler to examine the uterine arteries in 1757 singleton pregnancies attending for routine ultrasound examination at 23 weeks[17]. Increased impedance was observed in 7.3% of patients, including 5.1% with mean pulsatility index of more than 1.45 and 4.4% with bilateral notches. Increased pulsatility index identified 35.3% of women who later developed pre-eclampsia and 80% with pre-eclampsia requiring delivery before 34 weeks; the respective values for bilateral notches were 32.3% and 80%. The sensitivity of increased pulsatility index (PI) for delivery of an infant with birth weight below the 10th centile was 20.9% and 70% for birth weight below the 10th centile delivering before 34 weeks; the respective values for bilateral notches were 13.3% and 50%. These findings suggest that a one-stage color Doppler screening program at 23 weeks identifies most women who subsequently develop the serious complications of impaired placentation associated with delivery before 34 weeks. The screening results are similar if the high-risk group is defined either as those with increased PI or those with bilateral notches.

Randomized controlled trial

Davies *et al.* randomized 2600 unselected women to Doppler and non-Doppler groups[18]. The Doppler studies were performed at 19–22 weeks and then at 32 weeks, unless the women were classified as being at high risk, in which case the Doppler studies were performed monthly. Continuous wave Doppler was used to obtain flow velocity waveforms in the lower lateral border of the uterus and an abnormal result was defined by the presence of an abnormal waveform bilaterally. There was a high frequency of pregnancy complications in women with abnormal uterine artery waveforms and it was concluded that abnormal waveforms are an indicator of subsequent fetal compromise. However, no improvement in neonatal outcome was demonstrated by routine Doppler screening.

PROPHYLAXIS STUDIES

Aspirin

Studies in the 1980s have suggested that low-dose aspirin in high-risk women reduces the prevalence of intrauterine growth restriction and pre-eclampsia[19–22]. However, a series of randomized studies have shown no effect on the complications[23–27]. In most studies, there were no adverse effects from aspirin, but in one study the incidence of antenatal, intrapartum and postpartum bleeding was increased[26]. The results of the randomized studies have been criticized because the women examined were mostly at low risk for placental insufficiency.

Three randomized studies have examined the value of prophylactic aspirin in women considered to be at high risk of pre-eclampsia and intrauterine growth restriction because they had increased impedance in the uterine arteries (Table 6)[28–30].

McParland *et al.* carried out a two-stage Doppler screening study of the uterine arteries at 18–20 weeks and again at 24 weeks[28]. Those with persistently high resistance index (more than 0.58) were randomized to aspirin (75 mg/day) versus placebo for the remainder of the pregnancy. The difference between the aspirin and placebo groups in the frequency of pregnancy-induced hypertension (13% vs. 25%) did not achieve significance, but there were significant differences in the frequencies of pre-eclampsia (2% vs. 19%) and hypertension occurring before 37 weeks of gestation (0% vs. 17%). Fewer aspirin-treated than placebo-treated women had low birth weight babies (15% vs. 25%), but this difference was not significant. The only perinatal death in the aspirin group followed a cord accident during labor, whereas the three perinatal deaths in the placebo group were all due to severe hypertensive disease. No maternal or neonatal side-effects were observed in either group.

Table 6 Randomized studies examining the value of prophylactic aspirin in women considered to be at high risk of pre-eclampsia and intrauterine growth restriction (GR) because they had increased impedance to flow in the uterine arteries

Study	n	Aspirin	Outcome	
McParland et al., 1990[28]	100	75 mg/day	pre-eclampsia:	aspirin 2%, placebo 19%
			GR (< 2.5 kg):	aspirin 15%, placebo 25% (NS)
Bower et al., 1996[29]	60	60 mg/day	severe pre-eclampsia:	aspirin 13%, placebo 38%
			GR (< 3rd centile):	aspirin 26%, placebo 41% (NS)
Morris et al., 1996[30]	102	100 mg/day	pre-eclampsia:	aspirin 8%, placebo 14% (NS)
			GR (< 10th centile):	aspirin 27%, placebo 22% (NS)

NS, not significant

Bower et al. carried out a two-stage Doppler screening study of the uterine arteries at 18–22 weeks and again at 24 weeks[29]. Those with persistently high resistance index or an early diastolic notch were randomized to aspirin (60 mg/day) or placebo. There was no significant difference in the incidence of intrauterine growth restriction (aspirin 26%, placebo 41%) or pre-eclampsia (aspirin 29%, placebo 41%), but severe pre-eclampsia (defined as a diastolic blood pressure of at least 110 mmHg with proteinuria of at least 300 mg/24 h or pre-eclampsia requiring treatment with intravenous antihypertensives and anticonvulsants) was significantly lower in the aspirin group (13%) than in the placebo group (38%). There was only one perinatal death and this occurred in a woman taking placebo. It was concluded that, in high-risk pregnancy, low-dose aspirin commenced at 24 weeks may reduce the incidence of severe pre-eclampsia.

Morris et al. examined the uterine arteries by color Doppler at 18 weeks of gestation in 955 nulliparous women[30]. An abnormal result (defined by a high resistance index and the presence of an ipsilateral early diastolic notch) was found in 186 women, and 102 of these agreed to randomization to either low-dose aspirin (100 mg/day) or placebo for the remainder of the pregnancy. Abnormal uterine artery flow velocity waveforms were associated with statistically significant increases in pre-eclampsia (11 vs. 4%), birth weight below the tenth centile (28 vs. 11%), and adverse pregnancy outcome (45 vs. 28%). Prophylactic aspirin therapy did not result in a significant reduction in pregnancy complications. It was concluded that, although abnormal uteroplacental resistance at 18 weeks of gestation is associated with a significant increase in adverse pregnancy outcome, low-dose aspirin does not reduce pregnancy complications in women with uteroplacental insufficiency.

Antioxidants

Impaired placental perfusion is thought to stimulate the release of pre-eclamptic factors that enter the maternal circulation and cause vascular endothelial dysfunction. Free oxygen radicals are possible promoters of maternal vascular dysfunction. It was, therefore, hypothesized that early supplementation with antioxidants may be effective in decreasing oxidative stress and improving vascular endothelial function, thereby preventing, or ameliorating, the course of pre-eclampsia[31].

Chappell et al. identified 283 women as being at increased risk of pre-eclampsia by abnormal two-stage uterine artery Doppler analysis or a previous history of the disorder[32]. The patients were randomly assigned to vitamin C (1000 mg/day) and vitamin E (400 IU/day) or to placebo at 16–22 weeks of gestation. In the intention-to-treat cohort, pre-eclampsia occurred significantly more commonly in the placebo group (17% of 142 women) than in the vitamin group (8% of 141). These findings suggest that supplementation with vitamins C and E may be beneficial in the prevention of pre-eclampsia in women at increased risk of the disease. Multicenter trials are needed to show whether vitamin supplementation affects the occurrence of pre-eclampsia in low-risk women and to confirm these results in larger groups of high-risk women from different populations.

Nitric oxide donors

Nitric oxide, produced by the endothelium of blood vessels, is a potent vasodilator and inhibitor of platelet aggregation. Pre-eclampsia is associated with impaired production or function of nitric oxide and there is some evidence that treatment with the nitric oxide donor, glyceryl trinitrate, may reduce the prevalence or severity of this complication.

Ramsay et al. examined 15 women with increased impedance in the uterine arteries (mean resistance index of more than 0.6 and bilateral notches) at 24–26 weeks[33]. Infusion of glyceryl trinitrate was associated with a dose-dependent reduction in impedance to flow in the uterine arteries without a significant change in blood pressure, pulse rate or impedance in the umbilical artery or maternal carotid arteries. Grunewald et al. gave glyceryl trinitrate intravenously to women with severe pre-eclampsia and reported a decrease in maternal blood pressure and impedance in the umbilical artery, with no change in the impedance to flow in the uterine arteries[34]. The effect of glyceryl trinitrate in this study may have been mediated by its placental transfer into the fetal vascular circuit, causing direct vasodilatation of the umbilical circulation. A similar effect has been shown using sublingual isosorbide dinitrate in healthy second-trimester pregnancy; umbilical and uterine artery impedances were lowered[35].

Lees *et al.* reported a randomized study of 40 women with abnormal uterine artery Doppler results at 24–26 weeks of gestation[36]. Women were randomly allocated to receive transdermal glyceryl trinitrate 5-mg patches per day or equivalent placebo patches for 10 weeks or until delivery. The rates of pre-eclampsia, fetal growth restriction or preterm delivery were not significantly different in the two groups. Furthermore, there were no significant differences in maternal systolic and diastolic blood pressure, mean uterine artery resistance index and fetal umbilical and midde cerebral artery PIs between the groups.

CONCLUSIONS

- Increased impedance to flow in the uterine arteries in both high-risk and low-risk pregnancies is associated with increased risk for subsequent development of pre-eclampsia and intrauterine growth restriction.

- Women with normal impedance to flow in the uterine arteries constitute a group that have a low risk of developing obstetric complications related to uteroplacental insufficiency.

- Increased impedance to flow in the uterine arteries at 24 weeks of gestation is found in about 5% of pregnancies attending for routine antenatal care. The prevalence of high impedance at 20 weeks is about 2–3 times higher than at 24 weeks.

- Increased impedance to flow in the uterine arteries in pregnancies attending for routine antenatal care identifies about 50% of those that subsequently develop pre-eclampsia. Abnormal Doppler is better in predicting severe rather than mild pre-eclampsia. The sensitivity for severe pre-eclampsia is about 75%.

- Increased impedance to flow in the uterine arteries in pregnancies attending for routine antenatal care identifies about 30% of those that subsequently develop intrauterine growth restriction. Abnormal Doppler is better in predicting severe (birth weight below the 3rd centile or growth restriction requiring delivery before 35 weeks) rather than mild growth restriction.

- In pregnancies with increased impedance to flow in the uterine arteries, prophylactic treatment with low-dose aspirin or vitamins C and E may reduce the risk for subsequent development of pre-eclampsia.

REFERENCES

1. Arduini D, Rizzo G, Romanini C, Mancuso S. Uteroplacental blood flow velocity waveforms as predictors of pregnancy-induced hypertension. *Eur J Obstet Gynaecol Reprod Biol* 1987;26:335–41

2. Jacobson S-L, Imhof R, Manning N, Mannion V, Little D, Rey E, Redman C. The value of Doppler assessment of the uteroplacental circulation in predicting preeclampsia or intrauterine growth retardation. *Am J Obstet Gynecol* 1990;162:110–14

3. Zimmermann P, Eirio V, Koskinen J, Kujansuu E, Ranta T. Doppler assessment of the uterine and uteroplacental circulation in the second trimester in pregnancies at high risk for pre-eclampsia and/or intrauterine growth retardation: comparison and correlation between different Doppler parameters. *Ultrasound Obstet Gynecol* 1997;9:330–8

4. Campbell S, Pearce JM, Hackett G, Cohen-Overbeek T, Hernandez C. Qualitative assessment of uteroplacental blood flow: early screening test for high-risk pregnancies. *Obstet Gynecol* 1986;68: 649–53

5. Hanretty KP, Primrose MH, Neilson JP, Whittle MJ. Pregnancy screening by Doppler utero-placental and umbilical artery waveforms. *Br J Obstet Gynaecol* 1989;96:1163–7

6. Bewley S, Cooper D, Campbell S. Doppler investigation of uteroplacental blood flow resistance in the second trimester: a screening study for pre-eclampsia and intrauterine growth retardation. *Br J Obstet Gynaecol* 1991;98:871–9

7. Bower S, Schuchter K, Campbell S. Doppler ultrasound screening as part of routine antenatal scanning: prediction of pre-eclampsia and intrauterine growth retardation. *Br J Obstet Gynaecol* 1993;100:989–94

8. Valensise H, Bezzeccheri V, Rizzo G, Tranquilli AL, Garzetti GG, Romanini C. Doppler velocimetry of the uterine artery as a screening test for gestational hypertension. *Ultrasound Obstet Gynecol* 1993;3:18–22

9. North RA, Ferrier C, Long D, Townend K, Kincaid-Smith P. Uterine artery Doppler flow velocity waveforms in the second trimester for the prediction of preeclampsia and fetal growth retardation. *Obstet Gynecol* 1994;83:378–86

10. Chan FY, Pun TC, Lam C, Khoo J, Lee CP, Lam YH. Pregnancy screening by uterine artery Doppler velocimetry – which criterion performs best? *Obstet Gynecol* 1995;85:596–602

11. Irion O, Masse J, Forest JC, Moutquin JM. Prediction of pre-eclampsia, low birthweight for gestation and prematurity by uterine artery blood flow velocity waveforms analysis in low risk nulliparous women. *Br J Obstet Gynaecol* 1998;105:422–9

12. Kurdi W, Campbell S, Aquilina J, England P, Harrington K. The role of color Doppler imaging of the uterine arteries at 20 weeks' gestation in stratifying antenatal care. *Ultrasound Obstet Gynecol* 1998;12:339–45

13. Steel SA, Pearce JM, McParland P, Chamberlain GV. Early Doppler ultrasound screening in prediction of hypertensive disorders of pregnancy. *Lancet* 1990;335:1548–51

14. Bower S, Bewley S, Campbell S. Improved prediction of pre-eclampsia by two-stage screening of uterine arteries using the early diastolic notch and color Doppler imaging. *Obstet Gynecol* 1993;82: 78–83

15. Harrington K, Cooper D, Lees C, Hecher K, Campbell S. Doppler ultrasound of the uterine arteries: the importance of bilateral notching in the prediction of pre-eclampsia, placental abruption or delivery of a small-for-gestational-age baby. *Ultrasound Obstet Gynecol* 1996;7:182–8

16. Frusca T, Soregaroli M, Valcamonico A, Guandalini F, Danti L. Doppler velocimetry of the uterine arteries in nulliparous women. *Early Hum Dev* 1997;48:177–85

17. Albaiges G, Missfelder-Lobos H, Lees C, Parra M, Nicolaides KH. One-stage screening for pregnancy complications by color Doppler assessment of the uterine arteries at 23 weeks' gestation. *Obstet Gynecol* 2000;in press

18. Davies JA, Gallivan S, Spencer JAD. Randomised controlled trial of Doppler ultrasound screening of placental perfusion during pregnancy. *Lancet* 1992;340:1299–303

19. Beaufils M, Uzan S, Donsimoni R, Colau JC. Prevention of pre-eclampsia by early antiplatelet therapy. *Lancet* 1985;1:840–2

20. Wallenburg HCS, Dekker GA, Makovitz JW, Rotmans P. Low-dose aspirin prevents pregnancy-induced hypertension and pre-eclampsia in angiotensin-sensitive primigravidae. *Lancet* 1986;1:1–3

21. Schiff E, Peleg E, Goldenberg M, *et al*. The use of aspirin to prevent pregnancy induced hypertension and lower the ratio of thromboxane A2 to prostacyclin in relatively high risk pregnancies. *N Engl J Med* 1989;321:351–6

22. Uzan S, Beaufils M, Breart G, *et al*. Prevention of fetal growth retardation with low dose aspirin: findings of the EPREDA trial. *Lancet* 1991;337:1427–31

23. Italian Study of Aspirin in Pregnancy. Low-dose aspirin in prevention and treatment of intrauterine growth retardation and pregnancy-induced hypertension. *Lancet* 1993;341:396–400

24. CLASP (Collaborative Low-dose Aspirin Study in Pregnancy) Collaborative Group. CLASP: a randomised trial of low-dose aspirin for the prevention and treatment of pre-eclampsia among 9364 pregnant women. *Lancet* 1994;343:619

25. Sibai BM, Caritis SN, Thom E, *et al*. Prevention of preeclampsia with low-dose aspirin in healthy, nulliparous pregnant women. The National Institute of Child Health and Human Development Network of Maternal–Fetal Medicine Units. *N Engl J Med* 1993;329:1213–18

26. Golding J. A randomised trial of low dose aspirin for primiparae in pregnancy. The Jamaica Low Dose Aspirin Study Group. *Br J Obstet Gynaecol* 1998;105:293–9

27. Caritis S, Sibai B, Hauth J, *et al*. Low dose aspirin to prevent pre-eclampsia in women at high risk. *N Engl J Med* 1998;338:701–5

28. McParland P, Pearce JM, Chamberlain GV. Doppler ultrasound and aspirin in recognition and prevention of pregnancy-induced hypertension. *Lancet* 1990;335:1552–5

29. Bower SJ, Harrington KF, Schuchter K, McGirr C, Campbell S. Prediction of pre-eclampsia by abnormal uterine Doppler ultrasound and modification by aspirin. *Br J Obstet Gynaecol* 1996;103:625–9

30. Morris JM, Fay RA, Ellwood DA, Cook CM, Devonald KJ. A randomized controlled trial of aspirin in patients with abnormal uterine artery blood flow. *Obstet Gynecol* 1996;87:74–8

31. Schiff E, Friedman SA, Stampfer M, Kao L, Barrett PH, Sibai BM. Dietary consumption and plasma concentrations of vitamin E in pregnancies complicated by preeclampsia. *Am J Obstet Gynecol* 1996;175:1024–8

32. Chappell LC, Seed PT, Briley AL, Kelly FJ, Lee R, Hunt BJ, Parmar K, Bewley SJ, Shennan AH, Steer PJ, Poston L. Effect of antioxidants on the occurrence of pre-eclampsia in women at increased risk: a randomised trial. *Lancet* 1999;354:810–16

33. Ramsay B, de Belder A, Campbell S, Moncada S, Martin JF. A nitric oxide donor improves uterine artery diastolic blood flow in normal early pregnancy and in women at high risk of pre-eclampsia. *Eur J Clin Invest* 1994;24:76–8

34. Grunewald C, Kublickas M, Carlstrom K, Lunell N-O, Nisell H. Effects of nitroglycerin on the uterine and umbilical circulation in severe preeclampsia. *Obstet Gynecol* 1995;86:600–4

35. Thaler I, Amit A, Jakobi P, *et al.* The effect of isosorbide dinitrate on uterine artery and umbilical artery flow velocity waveforms at mid-pregnancy. *Obstet Gynecol* 1996;88:838–43

36. Lees C, Valensise H, Black R, Harrington K, Byers S, Romanini C, Campbell S. The efficacy and fetal-maternal cardiovascular effects of transdermal glyceryl trinitrate in the prophylaxis of pre-eclampsia and its complications: a randomized double-blind placebo-controlled trial. *Ultrasound Obstet Gynecol* 1998;12:334–8

6

Doppler studies in red blood cell isoimmunization

PATHOPHYSIOLOGY

In red cell isoimmunized pregnancies, maternal hemolytic antibodies cross the placenta and attach themselves onto fetal red cells, which are then destroyed in the fetal reticulo-endothelial system[1]. In mild to moderate disease there is a compensatory increase in intramedullary erythropoiesis, and in severe disease there is recruitment of extramedullary erythropoietic sites, such as liver and spleen[2,3].

Fetal blood pO_2, pCO_2 and pH usually remain within the normal range except in extreme anemia, when hypoxia and acidosis occur[4,5]. The fetal blood oxygen content decreases in proportion to the degree of anemia. The fetal 2,3-diphosphoglycerate (2,3-DPG) concentration is increased and the consequent decrease in hemoglobin–oxygen affinity presumably improves delivery of oxygen to the tissues[6]. In moderate anemia, the umbilical arterial plasma lactate concentration is increased but this is cleared by a single passage of fetal blood through the placenta and normal umbilical venous levels are maintained[7]. In severe anemia, when the oxygen content is less than 2 mmol/l, the placental capacity for lactate clearance is exceeded and the umbilical venous concentration increases exponentially. These data suggest that, in the fetus, systemic metabolic acidosis can be prevented, unless the oxygen content decreases below the critical level of 2 mmol/l[7]. When the fetal hemoglobin concentration deficit exceeds 6 g/dl, hydrops fetalis develops[1]. This may be the result of extensive infiltration of the liver by erythropoietic tissue, leading to portal hypertension, due to parenchymal compression of portal vessels, and hypoproteinemia, due to impaired protein synthesis[8]. Furthermore, at this hemoglobin concentration deficit, the oxygen content decreases below the critical level of 2 mmol/l.

DIAGNOSIS AND TREATMENT OF FETAL ANEMIA

The severity of fetal hemolysis can be predicted from:

(1) The history of previously affected pregnancies;

(2) The level of maternal hemolytic antibodies;

(3) Changes in the flow velocity waveforms obtained by Doppler studies of the fetal circulation;

(4) The altered morphometry of fetus and placenta; and

(5) The presence of pathological fetal heart rate patterns[4].

However, there is a wide scatter of values around the regression lines describing the associations between the degree of fetal anemia and the data obtained from these indirect methods of assessment.

The only accurate method for determining the severity of the disease is blood sampling by cordocentesis and measurement of the fetal hemoglobin concentration. Cordocentesis should be performed for all patients with a history of severe disease and those with a hemolytic antibody level of more than 15 IU/ml or a titer of 1 in 128 or more[9–12].

At cordocentesis, a fetal blood sample is first obtained and the hemoglobin concentration is determined. If this is below the normal range, the tip of the needle is kept in the lumen of the umbilical cord vessel and fresh, packed, rhesus-negative blood compatible with that of the mother is infused manually into the fetal circulation through a 10-ml syringe or a transfusion set. At the end of the transfusion, a further fetal blood sample is aspirated to determine the final hemoglobin concentration[13,14].

Subsequent transfusions are given at 1–3-weekly intervals until 34–36 weeks, and their timing is based on the findings of non-invasive tests, such as Doppler studies, and the knowledge that, following a fetal blood transfusion, the mean rate of decrease in fetal hemoglobin is approximately 0.3 g/dl per day[14].

DOPPLER STUDIES

Uterine artery

In a longitudinal study of 12 fetuses, Copel *et al.* included the uterine artery pulsatility index (PI), together with the descending thoracic aortic peak velocity, in a multiple regression model to predict whether the fetal hematocrit was below or above 25% before the second fetal blood transfusion[15]. The authors suggested that the significant contribution of uterine artery PI to the model could be explained by the effect of resolving placental edema after the correction of fetal anemia by the second transfusion. However, this is unlikely because there was no difference in uterine PI between hydropic and non-hydropic fetuses.

In a series of 95 red cell isoimmunized pregnancies, impedance in the uterine artery was within the normal range and there was no significant association between PI and the degree of fetal anemia[16]. Therefore, it is unlikely that fetal anemia alters the uteroplacental circulation.

Umbilical artery

Rightmire *et al.* found a significant inverse correlation between impedance to flow in the umbilical artery and fetal hematocrit[17]. It was suggested that increased impedance to flow in the fetoplacental microcirculation may be due to hypoxemia-mediated capillary endothelial cell damage, or clogging of the placental capillaries by the large fetal erythroblasts.

In contrast, Warren *et al.* reported that impedance in the umbilical artery was not abnormal in red cell isoimmunized pregnancies with high amniotic fluid bilirubin concentration[18]. Similarly, in a study of 95 affected pregnancies, umbilical artery PI, measured immediately before cordocentesis, was not increased and was not associated with fetal anemia[16].

Impedance to flow in fetal vessels

Vyas *et al.* measured the PI in the middle cerebral artery of 24 non-hydropic fetuses from red cell isoimmunized pregnancies; there were no significant associations between PI and either the degree of fetal anemia or the degree of deficit in oxygen content measured in samples obtained by cordocentesis[12]. Furthermore, in a study of 95 fetuses undergoing cordocentesis for rhesus disease, the PI in both the middle cerebral artery and descending thoracic aorta was not significantly different from normal controls and there was no significant association between PI and fetal anemia[16]. These findings indicate that impedance to flow is not affected by anemic hypoxia and by the alterations of blood constituents, such as hypoproteinemia, or red cell morphology, such as erythroblastemia, that accompany severe anemia[2,3].

Fetal cardiac Doppler studies

Meijboom *et al.* measured maximal and mean temporal velocity and early passive to late active ventricular filling phase (E/A) ratio on the atrioventricular orifices in 12 fetuses immediately before fetal blood transfusion[19]. There was a non-significant increase in both maximal and mean temporal velocities. Furthermore, there was a significant reversal in the E/A ratio in the flow waveforms from the tricuspid valve. In normal fetuses, these two peaks present an 'M' shape, whereas in anemic fetuses the E peak is dominant, suggesting that, in fetal anemia, there is an increased pre-load in the right atrium.

Copel *et al.* found that anemic fetuses before any intrauterine transfusion had significantly higher stroke volumes and ventricular outputs than normal controls. The increase was shared proportionately by both ventricles[20]. However, there was no significant relationship between fetal hematocrit and cardiac output. Nevertheless, extremely compromised fetuses demonstrated diminished cardiac function as a terminal finding. In contrast, Barss *et al.* reported a case of hydrops fetalis where the cardiac output measured before an intravascular transfusion was close to the normal mean for gestation[21].

Rizzo *et al.* measured right and left cardiac outputs (by multiplying the tricuspid or mitral mean temporal velocities, valvular area and heart rate) in 12 anemic fetuses before blood transfusion by cordocentesis[22]. Both left and right cardiac outputs were significantly higher for gestation than in 187 normal controls. Furthermore, the E/A ratios of both atrioventricular valves were higher than normal (Figure 1).

Lam *et al.* examined 20 anemic (due to homozygous α-thalassemia-1) fetuses at 12–13 weeks of gestation and reported increased peak velocities at the pulmonary valve and ascending aorta and an increased inner diameter of the pulmonary valve[23]. The total cardiac output was increased by one-third and this was mainly due to an increase of the cardiac output on the right side.

The findings of increased fetal cardiac output in anemia are in agreement with the results of animal studies and confirm the prediction, from a mathematical model, that, in fetal anemia, the cardiac output is increased to maintain an adequate oxygen delivery to the tissues[24]. Possible mechanisms include, first, decreased blood viscosity leading to

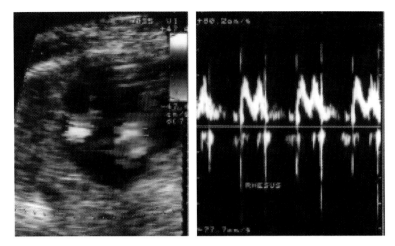

Figure 1 Flow velocity waveforms across the tricuspid valve in an anemic fetus at 28 weeks of gestation. The E/A ratio is increased (0.97 compared to the expected mean for gestation of 0.75)

increased venous return and cardiac preload and, second, peripheral vasodilatation as a result of a fall in blood oxygen content and therefore reduced cardiac afterload. The high E/A is suggestive of increased cardiac preload. Since right-to-left cardiac output ratio is normal, there is no evidence of redistribution in cardiac output similar to that described in hypoxemic growth-restricted fetuses. These findings suggest that, in fetal anemia, the changes in fetal cardiac output are mainly due to low blood viscosity. An alternative explanation is that the symmetrical increase in cardiac output is secondary to an increase in catecholamine concentrations in fetal blood induced by anemia[25].

Blood velocity in fetal arteries

Rightmire et al. examined 21 fetuses from red cell isoimmunized pregnancies before fetal blood sampling and reported a significant inverse association between aortic mean blood velocity and fetal hemoglobin concentration[17]. Similarly, from the examination of 68 previously untransfused fetuses at 17–37 weeks of gestation, Nicolaides et al. reported a significant association between aortic mean velocity, measured immediately before cordocentesis, and the degree of fetal anemia[11]. However, separate analysis of non-hydropic and hydropic fetuses demonstrated that in the former group there was a significant positive correlation between increased velocity and fetal anemia, whilst in the latter group there was a significant negative correlation between these two parameters. In an extended series of 95 previously untransfused fetuses undergoing cordocentesis for rhesus disease, there was a significant increase in aortic velocity with the degree of fetal anemia[16]. Although, in some hydropic fetuses, aortic velocity was decreased, in the majority of cases the velocity was increased. In an additional series of

212 fetuses that had a transfusion 2–3 weeks previously, the relation between aortic velocity and anemia was weaker.

Copel *et al.* measured the peak velocity in 16 fetuses immediately before cordocentesis and derived a series of formulae for the prediction of whether the fetal hematocrit was above or below 25%[15]. The best prediction was achieved for the untransfused fetuses. For subsequent transfusions, different formulae had to be used, presumably because of the different rheological properties of adult, rather than fetal, blood in the fetal circulation.

Bilardo *et al.* measured mean velocity in the common carotid artery of 12 previously untransfused anemic fetuses immediately before cordocentesis[26]. There was a significant association between the degree of fetal anemia and the increase in blood velocity. The authors speculated that this increase in common carotid artery velocity reflected increased cardiac output associated with fetal anemia, rather than a chemoreceptor-mediated redistribution in blood flow, as seen in hypoxemic growth-restricted fetuses[27].

Vyas *et al.*, in a study of 24 previously untransfused, non-hydropic fetuses from red cell isoimmunized pregnancies at 18–35 weeks of gestation, reported a significant correlation between an increase in mean velocity in the middle cerebral artery and the degree of fetal anemia measured in samples obtained by cordocentesis[12]. In an extended series of 95 previously untransfused fetuses undergoing cordocentesis for rhesus disease, there was a significant association between the increase in mean velocity in the middle cerebral artery with the degree of fetal anemia[16]. In an additional series of 212 fetuses that had a transfusion 2–3 weeks previously, the relation between blood velocity and anemia was weaker[16].

Mari *et al.* found a significant association between the peak systolic velocity in the middle cerebral artery and fetal hematocrit at cordocentesis. In a prospective study of 16 fetuses from isoimmunized pregnancies, they found that all the anemic fetuses had peak velocity values above the normal mean for gestation, whereas none of the fetuses with peak velocity below the normal mean was anemic[28]. On the basis of these results, they suggested that, in the management of isoimmunized pregnancies, the indication for cordocentesis should be a peak systolic velocity above the normal mean for gestation. These results were confirmed in a multicenter study involving 111 fetuses from isoimmunized pregnancies; all moderately or severely anemic fetuses had increased peak velocity in the middle cerebral artery[29].

Steiner *et al.* performed 112 fetal blood samplings by cordocentesis in 33 cases with rhesus isoimmunization and found that the mean peak systolic aortic velocity of anemic fetuses was significantly higher than that of unaffected fetuses[30]. Furthermore, there was a good correlation between delta peak velocities and delta hematocrits for the first procedure.

Bahado-Singh *et al.* examined the main splenic artery waveforms in 22 non-hydropic fetuses from red cell isoimmunized pregnancies[31]. The deceleration angle between the line describing the average slope during the diastolic phase of the cycle and the vertical axis was measured and expressed in multiples of the median (MoM) for gestational age. A decrease in the deceleration angle was associated with fetal anemia and, at a threshold deceleration angle of < 0.60 MoM, the sensitivity for severe anemia (hemoglobin deficit of 5 g/dl) was 100%, with an 8.8% false-positive rate. It was concluded that all cases of severe anemia could be identified before the development of hydrops, and, if, in the management of red cell isoimmunization, cordocentesis is only carried out if the deceleration angle is < 0.60 MoM, then the need for cordocentesis would decrease by more than 90%[31].

The findings of increased blood velocity in the fetal arteries with anemia (Figures 2 and 3) are compatible with the data from the fetal cardiac Doppler studies. If it is assumed that, in anemia, the cross-sectional area of the fetal descending aorta and middle cerebral arteries does not change, the increased velocity would reflect an increase in both central and peripheral blood flow due to increased cardiac output. The decreased aortic velocity in some hydropic fetuses may be the consequence of cardiac

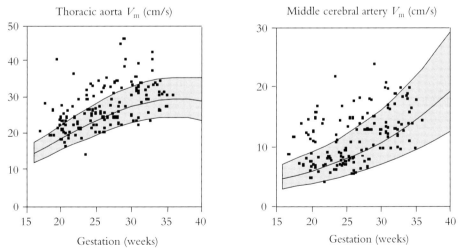

Figure 2   Blood velocity in the fetal thoracic aorta (left) and middle cerebral artery (right) in red cell isoimmunized pregnancies plotted on the appropriate reference range (mean, 95th and 5th centiles) for gestation. Fetal anemia is associated with a hyperdynamic circulation

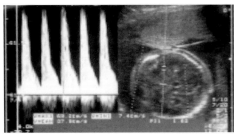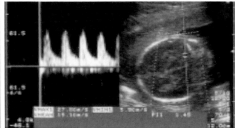

Figure 3   Flow velocity waveform in the fetal middle cerebral artery in a severely anemic fetus at 22 weeks (left) and in a normal fetus (right). In fetal anemia, blood velocity is increased

decompensation, presumably due to the associated hypoxia and lactic acidosis and to the impaired venous return due to liver infiltration with hemopoietic tissue[2].

Blood velocity in fetal veins

Rightmire *et al.* measured the fetal inferior vena caval time averaged mean velocity immediately before the first intravascular fetal blood transfusion in 19 rhesus-affected pregnancies at 18–28 weeks of gestation[17]. Although the velocity was higher than in non-anemic controls, there was no significant correlation with fetal hematocrit. In the same study, the intrahepatic umbilical venous velocity was not significantly different from non-anemic controls.

In contrast, Kirkinen *et al.* examined 18 rhesus isoimmunized pregnancies within 4 days before delivery and reported that, in anemic fetuses, the volume flow in the intrahepatic umbilical vein was significantly increased due to both increased blood velocity and vessel diameter[32]. Similarly, Warren *et al.* performed serial measurements of fetal blood flow in 51 rhesus isoimmunized pregnancies and reported that increased flow was associated with subsequent development of fetal hydrops or rise in amniotic fluid bilirubin concentration[18]. It was postulated that the increased flow was the result of reduced blood viscosity due to the reduced hematocrit.

Iskaros *et al.* performed serial measurements of umbilical vein maximal flow velocity and found that elevated velocities prior to delivery were predictive of the need for exchange blood transfusion[33]. They concluded that pregnancies with a mild or no history of fetal anemia may be monitored by a combination of serial antibody quantification and Doppler measurement of umbilical vein maximal flow velocities.

Oepkes *et al.*, in a study of 21 previously transfused fetuses from red cell isoimmunized pregnancies, reported increased peak systolic and time averaged maximum velocities in the ductus venosus before intravascular fetal blood transfusion, which returned to normal values the following day[34]. It was suggested that the increase in ductus venosus blood flow in anemic fetuses reflects increased venous return and therefore cardiac preload.

Hecher *et al.* recorded flow velocity waveforms from the ductus venosus, right hepatic vein, inferior vena cava, middle cerebral artery and descending thoracic aorta from 38 red cell isoimmunized pregnancies and found that only the velocity in the thoracic aorta was significantly associated with the degree of fetal anemia[35]. Furthermore, this study showed that heart failure is not the primary mechanism for the development of hydrops, but rather the end-stage of severe anemia, because the pulsatility of venous blood flow waveforms was not increased. Hydrops may be due to reduced colloid osmotic pressure, hypoxia–induced endothelial damage and increased permeability.

Severe fetal anemia, with consequent cardiac failure, is associated with a reversed 'a' wave in the ductus venosus. Under these conditions, pulsations are also present in the venous portal system (which in normal fetuses is characterized by a continuous flow). The pulsatile pattern present in the venous system corresponds to findings in children with portal hypertension[36].

Since, in fetal anemia, resistance to flow in the fetal circulation and placenta is unchanged, an increase of umbilical venous blood flow is in accordance with high cardiac output and elevated arterial velocities.

Hemodynamic changes following fetal blood transfusion

Warren *et al.* and Kirkinen *et al.* found that, immediately after a fetal *intraperitoneal blood transfusion*, there was a temporary increase in umbilical venous blood flow and subsequent gradual decrease from above to within the normal range[18,32]. It was suggested that the gradual decrease in flow, coinciding with resolution of fetal ascites, was the result of absorption of the transfused blood and correction of the fetal anemia.

Copel *et al.* measured impedance to flow in the uterine and umbilical arteries and peak velocity in the descending thoracic aorta immediately before and 12 hours after fetal blood *exchange transfusion* by cordocentesis; no differences were found[15].

Doppler studies of impedance to flow in the umbilical artery before and soon after intravascular *top-up transfusion* provided conflicting results. In a study of 43 cases, Bilardo *et al.* found no significant changes[26]. In contrast, Weiner and Anderson and Hanretty *et al.* reported a significant decrease in impedance immediately after fetal blood transfusion in 19 and 22 fetuses, respectively[37,38]. It was postulated that simple needling of fetal blood vessels stimulates a humoral vasodilator mechanism. Supportive evidence was provided by the finding that fetal blood levels of vasoactive substances with vasodilatatory effects, like prostaglandins and atrial natriuretic peptide, are increased after an intravascular blood transfusion[39,40]. However, as Welch et al. pointed out, the possible changes in indices of impedance after an intrauterine transfusion may not be simply due to vasodilatation but due to the complex influences of altered fetal whole blood viscosity, increased number of scattering particles (red cells) and vasoactive compounds[41].

Bilardo et al. performed fetal Doppler studies in 43 cases immediately before and within 30 minutes of an intravascular top-up transfusion[26]. There was a significant decrease in mean blood velocity in both the descending thoracic aorta (Figure 4) and common carotid artery. Similarly, Mari et al. found that intrauterine transfusion is associated with a significant decrease in the peak velocity in the middle cerebral artery and this decrease is proportional to the increase in fetal hematocrit[42]. These findings are likely to be the result of a decrease in cardiac output following the transfusion due to:

(1) Increased blood hemoglobin concentration and viscosity, and consequent decrease in venous return;

(2) Congestive heart failure due to overloading of the fetal circulation; or

(3) Cardio-inhibition due to increased baroreceptor activity.

Confirmatory evidence of a decrease in cardiac output following blood transfusion was provided by Rizzo et al.[22]. They measured left and right cardiac outputs before and at 15-min intervals for 2 hours after an intravascular top-up transfusion in 12 fetuses. After transfusion, there was a significant temporary fall in both right and left cardiac outputs. Furthermore, the E/A ratios in both the tricuspid and mitral valves were increased suggesting that cardiac preload was also increased. Within 2 hours after transfusion, both parameters had returned towards the normal range. The fall in cardiac output was significantly related to the amount of expansion of the fetoplacental volume due to the transfusion. The most likely explanation for these findings is that transfusion results in temporary cardiovascular overload. Animal studies have also shown that the fetal heart has very limited reserve capacity to increase its output in response to acute overload, and that massive increases in fetal blood volume are associated with a decrease in cardiac output. After transfusion, there is a rapid rate of fluid loss and this explains the rapid recovery in E/A ratios and cardiac output[43].

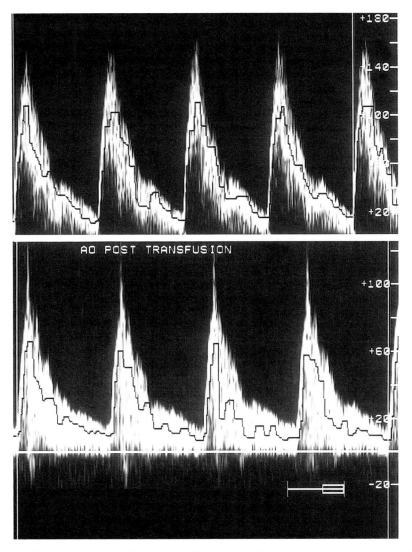

Figure 4 Flow velocity waveform in the fetal descending thoracic aorta in an anemic fetus demonstrating high velocities and Doppler 'window' for low velocities during systole (top). After blood transfusion, there is a decrease in peak systolic velocity and the Doppler 'window' has disappeared (bottom)

The short-lived nature of the hemodynamic effects of intravascular transfusion can also explain the findings of Mari *et al.* who reported that the middle cerebral artery PI, internal carotid artery PI and umbilical artery PI before and the day after fetal transfusion were not significantly different[44]. Similarly, Copel *et al.*, in a study of cardiac output at 12 hours after intravascular blood transfusion, found no significant differences from the pretransfusion levels[20].

CONCLUSIONS

- In red cell isoimmunized pregnancies, placentation is normal and therefore indices of impedance to flow in the uterine and umbilical arteries are normal, irrespective of the severity of fetal anemia.

- In red cell isoimmunized pregnancies, normal placental perfusion results in normal fetal blood pO_2, pCO_2 and pH and therefore there is no evidence of redistribution in the fetal circulation; the PI in the middle cerebral artery, thoracic aorta and renal arteries is normal.

- In red cell isoimmunized pregnancies, the left and right cardiac outputs and blood velocity in the umbilical vein, middle cerebral artery, thoracic aorta, renal arteries and the fetal venous system are increased in proportion to the degree of fetal anemia. The most likely mechanism for the hyperdynamic circulation of anemic fetuses is decreased blood viscosity, leading to increased venous return and cardiac preload.

- In red cell isoimmunized pregnancies, fetal heart failure is not the primary mechanism for the development of hydrops. However, severe anemia with consequent end-stage cardiac failure may be associated with high pulsatility or even reversed 'a' wave in the ductus venosus and pulsations in portal sinus.

- In red cell isoimmunized pregnancies, intravascular fetal blood transfusion results in temporary cardiovascular overload with a temporary fall in both right and left cardiac outputs.

REFERENCES

1. Nicolaides KH, Soothill PW, Clewell WH, Rodeck CH, Mibashan R, Campbell S. Fetal haemoglobin measurement in the assessment of red cell isoimmunization. *Lancet* 1988;i:1073–6

2. Nicolaides KH, Thilaganathan B, Rodeck CH, Mibashan RS. Erythroblastosis and reticulocytosis in anemic fetuses. *Am J Obstet Gynecol* 1988;159:1063–5

3. Nicolaides KH, Snijders RJM, Thorpe-Beeston JG, Van den Hof MC, Gosden CM, Bellingham AJ. Mean red cell volume in normal, small and anemic fetuses. *Fetal Therapy* 1989;4:1–13

4. Nicolaides KH. Studies on fetal physiology and pathophysiology in rhesus disease. *Semin Perinatol* 1989;13:328–37

5. Soothill PW, Nicolaides KH, Rodeck CH, Bellingham AJ. The effect of replacing fetal with adult hemoglobin on the blood gas and acid–base parameters in human fetuses. *Am J Obstet Gynecol* 1988; 158:66–9

6. Soothill PW, Lestas AN, Nicolaides KH, Rodeck CH, Bellingham AJ. 2,3-Diphosphoglycerate in normal, anaemic and transfused human fetuses. *Clin Sci* 1988;74:527–30

7. Soothill PW, Nicolaides KH, Rodeck CH, Clewell WH, Lindridge J. Relationship of fetal hemoglobin and oxygen content to lactate concentration in Rh isoimmunized pregnancies. *Obstet Gynecol* 1987;69:268–71

8. Nicolaides KH, Warenski JC, Rodeck CH. The relationship of fetal protein concentration and hemoglobin level to the development of hydrops in rhesus isoimmunization. *Am J Obstet Gynecol* 1985;152:341–4

9. Nicolaides KH, Rodeck CH. Maternal serum anti-D concentration in the assessment of rhesus isoimmunisation. *Br Med J* 2000;in press

10. Nicolaides KH, Sadovsky G, Cetin E. Fetal heart rate patterns in red blood cell isoimmunized pregnancies. *Am J Obstet Gynecol* 1989;161:351–6

11. Nicolaides KH, Bilardo CM, Campbell S. Prediction of fetal anemia by measurement of the mean blood velocity in the fetal aorta. *Am J Obstet Gynecol* 1990;162:209–12

12. Vyas S, Nicolaides KH, Campbell S. Doppler examination of the middle cerebral artery in anemic fetuses. *Am J Obstet Gynecol* 1990;162:1066–8

13. Nicolaides KH, Soothill PW, Rodeck CH, Campbell S. Ultrasound guided sampling of umbilical cord and placental blood to assess fetal wellbeing. *Lancet* 1986;i:1065–7

14. Nicolaides KH, Soothill PW, Rodeck CH, Clewell W. Rh disease: intravascular fetal blood transfusion by cordocentesis. *Fetal Therapy* 1986;1:185–92

15. Copel JA, Grannum PA, Belanger K, Green J, Hobbins JC. Pulsed Doppler flow velocity waveforms before and after intrauterine intravascular transfusion for severe erythroblastosis fetalis. *Am J Obstet Gynecol* 1988;158:768–74

16. Nicolaides KH, Kaminopetros P. Red-cell isoimmunization. In Pearce M, ed. *Doppler Ultrasound in Perinatal Medicine*. Oxford: Oxford University Press, 1992;244–57

17. Rightmire DA, Nicolaides KH, Rodeck CH, Campbell S. Fetal blood velocities in Rh isoimmunization: relationship to gestational age and to fetal hematocrit. *Obstet Gynecol* 1986;68:233–6

18. Warren PS, Gill RW, Fisher CC. Doppler blood flow studies in rhesus isoimmunization. *Sem Perinatol* 1987;11:375–8

19. Meijboom EJ, De Smedt MCH, Visser GHA, Jager W, Nicolaides KH. Fetal cardiac output measurements by Doppler echocardiography. In Proceedings of the *Sixth Annual Meeting of The Society of Perinatal Obstetricians*. San Antonio, Texas, 1986: Abstract 17

20. Copel JA, Grannum PA, Green JJ, Hobbins JC, Kleinman CS. Fetal cardiac output in the isoimmunized pregnancy: a pulsed Doppler echocardiographic study of patients undergoing intravascular intrauterine transfusion. *Am J Obstet Gynecol* 1989;161:361–4

21. Barss VA, Doubilet PM, St.John-Sutton M, Cartier MS, Frigoletto FD. Cardiac output in a fetus with erythrobastosis fetalis: assessment using pulsed Doppler. *Obstet Gynecol* 1987;70:442–4

22. Rizzo G, Nicolaides KH, Arduini D, Campbell S. Effects of intravascular fetal blood transfusion on fetal intracardiac Doppler velocity waveforms. *Am J Obstet Gynecol* 1990;163;569–71

23. Lam YH, Tang MH, Lee CP, Tse HY Cardiac blood flow studies in fetuses with homozygous alpha-thalassemia-1 at 12–13 weeks of gestation. *Ultrasound Obstet Gynecol* 1999;13:48–51

24. Huikeshoven FJ, Hope ID, Power GG, Gilbert RD, Longo LD. A comparison of sheep and human fetal oxygen delivery systems with use of a mathematical model. *Am J Obstet Gynecol* 1985;151:449–55

25. Oberhoffer R, Grab D, Keckstein J, Högel J, Terinde R, Lang D. Cardiac changes in fetuses secondary to immune hemolytic anemia and their relation to hemoglobin and catecholamine concentrations in fetal blood. *Ultrasound Obstet Gynecol* 1999;13:396–400

26. Bilardo CM, Nicolaides KH, Campbell S. Doppler studies in red cell isoimmunization. *Clin Obstet Gynecol* 1989;32:719–27

27. Bilardo CM, Nicolaides KH, Campbell S. Doppler measurements of fetal and utero-placental circulation: relationship with umbilical venous blood gases measured at cordocentesis. *Am J Obstet Gynecol* 1990;162:115–20.

28. Mari G, Adrignolo A, Abuhamad AZ, Pirhonen J, Jones DC, Ludomirsky A, Copel JA. Diagnosis of fetal anemia with Doppler ultrasound in the pregnancy complicated by maternal blood group immunization. *Ultrasound Obstet Gynecol* 1995;5:400–5

29. Mari G. Noninvasive diagnosis by Doppler ultrasonography of fetal anemia due to maternal red-cell alloimmunization. *N Engl J Med* 2000; 342: 9–14

30. Steiner H, Schaffer H, Spitzer D, Batka M, Graf AH, Staudach A. The relationship between peak velocity in the fetal descending aorta and hematocrit in rhesus isoimmunization. *Obstet Gynecol* 1995;85:659–62

31. Bahado-Singh R, Oz U, Deren O, Pirhonen J, Kovanci E, Copel J, Onderoglu L. A new splenic artery Doppler velocimetric index for prediction of severe fetal anemia associated with Rh alloimmunization. *Am J Obstet Gynecol* 1999;180:49–54

32. Kirkinen P, Jouppila P, Eik-Nes S. Umbilical vein blood flow in rhesus isoimmunization. *Br J Obstet Gynaecol* 1983;90:640–3

33. Iskaros J, Kingdom J, Morrison JJ, Rodeck C. Prospective non-invasive monitoring of pregnancies complicated by red cell alloimmunization. *Ultrasound Obstet Gynecol* 1998;11:432–7

34. Oepkes D, Vandenbussche FP, van Bel F, Kanhai HHH. Fetal ductus venosus blood flow velocities before and after transfusion in red-cell alloimmunized pregnancies. *Obstet Gynecol* 1993;82;237–41

35. Hecher K, Snijders R, Campbell S, Nicolaides K. Fetal venous, arterial, and intracardiac blood flows in red blood cell isoimmunization. *Obstet Gynecol* 1995;85:122–8

36. d'Ancona RL, Rahman F, Ozcan T, Copel JA, Mari G. The effect of intravascular blood transfusion on the flow velocity waveform of the portal venous system of the anemic fetus. *Ultrasound Obstet Gynecol* 1997; 10:333–7

37. Weiner CP, Anderson TL. The acute effect of cordocentesis with or without fetal curarization and of intravascular transfusion upon umbilical artery waveform indices. *Obstet Gynecol* 1989;73: 219–24

38. Hanretty KP, Whittle MJ, Gilmore DH, McNay MB, Howie CA, Rubin PC. The effect of intravascular transfusion for rhesus haemolytic disease on umbilical artery Doppler flow velocity waveforms. *Br J Obstet Gynaecol* 1989;96:960–3

39. Weiner CP, Robillard GE. Effect of acute intravascular volume expansion on human fetal prostaglandin concentrations. *Am J Obstet Gynecol* 1989;161:1494–7

40. Panos MZ, Nicolaides KH, Anderson JV, Economides DL, Rees L, Williams R. Plasma atrial natriuretic peptide: response to intravascular blood transfusion. *Am J Obstet Gynecol* 1989;161: 357–61

41. Welch CR, Rodeck CH. The effect of intravascular transfusion for rhesus haemolytic disease on umbilical artery Doppler flow velocity waveforms. *Br J Obstet Gynaecol* 1990;97:865–6

42. Mari G, Rahman F, Olofsson P, Ozcan T, Copel JA. Increase of fetal hematocrit decreases the middle cerebral artery peak systolic velocity in pregnancies complicated by rhesus allo-immunization. *J Matern Fetal Med* 1997;6:206–8

43. Gillbert RD. Control of fetal cardiac output during changes in blood volume. *Am J Physiol* 1980;238:H80–6

44. Mari G, Moise KJ, Russell LD, Kirshon B, Stefos T, Carpenter RJ. Flow velocity waveforms of the vascular system in the anemic fetus before and after intravascular transfusion for severe red blood cell alloimunization. *Am J Obstet Gynecol* 1990;162:1060–4

7

Doppler studies in pregnancies with maternal diabetes mellitus

PATHOPHYSIOLOGY

Maternal diabetes mellitus is associated with a high risk of fetal death. In the past, before the introduction of insulin, the main cause of death was in association with maternal keto-acidosis, but now most fetal deaths are non–keto-acidotic and occur in association with fetal macrosomia.

The major source of fetal glucose is the mother and there is a good correlation between maternal and fetal blood glucose concentrations[1]. In pregnancies complicated by diabetes mellitus, the maternal hyperglycemia causes fetal hyperglycemia and hyperinsulinemia[2,3]. Furthermore, the fetal insulin to glucose ratio is increased because hyperglycemia and/or the other metabolic derangements associated with maternal diabetes mellitus act on the fetal pancreas to cause β–cell hyperplasia and precocious pancreatic maturation[2]. Fetal hyperinsulinemia causes macrosomia, either directly through its anabolic effect on nutrient uptake and utilization, or indirectly through related peptides such as insulin-like growth factors[4].

Although good diabetic control in the third trimester of pregnancy reduces the incidence of macrosomia, the latter is not always preventable. In pregnant women with diabetes mellitus, despite stringent maternal glycemic control, the fluctuation in maternal glucose concentration is greater than in non–diabetics and it is possible that, during short-lived episodes of hyperglycemia, an already hyperplastic fetal pancreas will respond with a disproportionately high release of insulin.

In diabetic pregnancies, analysis of blood samples obtained by cordocentesis has demonstrated significant acidemia and hyperlacticemia in the absence of hypoxemia[5-7]. Fetal acidemia, which may offer an explanation for the unexplained stillbirths of

121

diabetic pregnancies, is likely to be the consequence of increased metabolic rate. Salvesen *et al.* performed cordocentesis in diabetic pregnancies and reported a significant association between fetal plasma insulin concentration and the degree of fetal acidemia[2]. In pregnant sheep, chronic hyperglycemia results in increased aerobic and anaerobic glucose metabolism, with consequent increased oxygen consumption, lactate production and fall in pH and pO_2[8-13]. Glucose oxidation and oxygen consumption are also increased by hyperinsulinemia, and this effect is independent of that caused by hyperglycemia[12]. Hyperlacticemia occurs because the fetus has a reduced capacity for oxidative metabolism and low pyruvate dehydrogenase activity. Severe hyperglycemia is characterized by acidemia and hypoxemia, but minor degrees of hyperglycemia are associated with acidemia in the absence of hypoxemia[8]. However, in the presence of mild fetal hypoxemia, minor degrees of fetal hyperglycemia do result in severe acidosis and even fetal death[13].

The alternative explanation for fetal acidemia in maternal diabetes mellitus is impaired placental perfusion. Histological studies have reported decreased villous surface area, villous edema and thickening of the basement membrane[14]. However, the finding that acidemia is not accompanied by hypoxemia suggests that the acidemia is unlikely to be due to impaired placental function; in pregnancies complicated by intrauterine growth restriction due to uteroplacental insufficiency, acidemia is accompanied by hypoxemia (see Chapter 4).

DOPPLER STUDIES OF THE UMBILICAL AND UTERINE ARTERIES

The aim of Doppler ultrasound studies of the umbilical and uterine arteries in diabetic pregnancies is to determine whether impedance to flow is related to maternal glycemic control and whether impedance is increased in patients with diabetic nephropathy and vasculopathy. This section also examines whether impedance in the uterine and umbilical arteries can provide useful prediction of subsequent development of pre-eclampsia and/or intrauterine growth restriction in the same way that it does in non-diabetic pregnancies.

Olofsson *et al.* examined 40 diabetic pregnancies and reported that the volume blood flow in the fetal aorta and umbilical vein and the pulsatility index (PI) in the umbilical artery were higher in diabetic than in non-diabetic pregnancies[15]. There was no significant association between these indices and the degree of diabetic control or fetal size, but the high umbilical artery PI and high aortic volume flow occurred in fetuses who later developed distress in labor. It was suggested that, in some diabetic pregnancies, there is increased placental vascular resistance with a compensatory increase in volume flow. A high umbilical artery PI cannot be considered characteristic of diabetic pregnancy, but fetal distress might be more common in diabetic pregnancy[15]. More recently, Ursem et al. examined 16 women with well-controlled insulin-dependent diabetes mellitus at 12–21 weeks of gestation and reported increased fetal heart rate variability and umbilical artery peak systolic velocity, but normal fetal heart rate and umbilical artery time-averaged velocity[16]. It was suggested that fetal heart rate variability and umbilical artery peak systolic velocity may be markers for fetal cardiovascular homeostasis in pregnancies complicated by insulin-dependent diabetes mellitus[16].

Bracero et al. performed Doppler studies of the umbilical artery during the third trimester of pregnancy in 43 women with diabetes mellitus[17]. They found a significant association between impedance to flow and maternal serum glucose concentration. Furthermore, high impedance was associated with an increased number of stillbirths and neonatal morbidity. It was suggested that maternal hyperglycemia causes placental vasoconstriction by impairing prostacyclin production[17]. In another study, Bracero et al. evaluated 207 singleton pregnancies complicated by maternal diabetes mellitus within 1 week of delivery. In 36% of cases, there was an adverse outcome (defined as delivery before 37 weeks, or fetal risk requiring Cesarean delivery, or fetal growth restriction, or neonatal hypocalcemia, hypoglycemia, hyperbilirubinemia, or respiratory distress syndrome)[18]. The relative risk of adverse outcome was 2.6 for increased impedance in the umbilical artery, which was higher than the risk of 1.7 for abnormal biophysical profile score or a non-reactive non-stress test[18]. Bracero et al. also measured impedance to flow in the left and right uterine arteries in 265 women with singleton pregnancies complicated by diabetes mellitus within 1 week before delivery[19]. The higher the difference in impedance between the two uterine arteries, the greater was the risk of adverse pregnancy outcome, but there was a considerable overlap in discordance between the good and adverse outcome groups.

Landon et al. performed serial measurements of impedance to flow in the umbilical artery in 35 insulin-dependent diabetic women, during the second and third trimesters, and found no significant association between this index and maternal blood glucose or glycosylated hemoglobin level[20]. Women with vascular disease had a higher impedance in the umbilical artery compared to those with uncomplicated diabetes. Increased impedance in women with vascular disease was associated with subsequent development of intrauterine growth restriction and, in those with no vascular disease, with the development of pre-eclampsia. Similarly, Dicker et al. carried out Doppler examinations of the umbilical artery in 108 pregnant women with insulin-dependent diabetes mellitus and found no significant association between impedance to flow and maternal blood glucose or glycosylated hemoglobin levels[21]. Increased umbilical artery impedance was associated with the subsequent development of pre-eclampsia (in women without vasculopathy) and development of intrauterine growth restriction in those with vasculopathy.

Reece *et al.* examined 56 diabetic pregnancies and reported that the umbilical artery PI was higher in patients with diabetic vasculopathy than in non-diabetic controls or in diabetic patients without vasculopathy. Intrauterine growth restriction and neonatal metabolic complications were also significantly correlated with elevated umbilical artery PI[22]. There was, however, no correlation between Doppler indices and maternal glucose values, although most were within a euglycemic range.

Ishimatsu *et al.* performed Doppler studies of the umbilical artery during the third trimester of pregnancy in 16 women with diabetes mellitus. They found no significant association between impedance to flow and maternal serum glucose or fructosamine levels[23]. However, in two patients with serum glucose levels of over 300 mg/dl, impedance was increased and returned to the normal range when the serum glucose level decreased to below 200 mg/dl.

Johnstone *et al.* measured impedance to flow in the umbilical artery in 128 pregnancies complicated by diabetes mellitus[24]. There was no significant association between impedance to flow and either short-term or long-term glycemic control. Although, in some cases that subsequently developed fetal distress, there was increased impedance, fetal compromise also occurred in association with normal impedance.

Zimmermann *et al.* carried out serial measurements of impedance to flow in the umbilical artery in 53 women with insulin-dependent diabetes. Impedance was within the normal range and there was no significant association with maternal blood glucose or glycosylated hemoglobin level or maternal vascular disease[25]. This group also measured impedance to flow in the uterine arteries in 43 pregnancies complicated by insulin-dependent diabetes mellitus and found no significant differences from normal or significant associations with short- and long-term glycemic control, maternal vasculopathy, or diabetes-specific fetal morbidity[26].

The effectiveness of screening for the complications of impaired placentation by uterine artery Doppler in diabetic pregnancies may be similar to that in non-diabetics[27]. Thus, Haddad *et al.* measured impedance to flow in the uterine arteries of 37 diabetic pregnancies and reported that increased impedance identified 45% of those that subsequently developed pre-eclampsia and/or intrauterine growth restriction. Barth *et al.* measured impedance to flow in the uterine arcuate artery system beneath the placenta within 8 days of delivery in 47 patients with insulin-dependent diabetes

Table 1 Doppler studies

Author	Doppler study	Diabetes vs. non-diabetes	Diabetic vasculopathy	Diabetic control
Olofsson et al., 1987[15]	umbilical	increased		no correlation
Bracero et al., 1986[17]	umbilical	increased		good correlation
Landon et al., 1989[20]	umbilical		increased	no correlation
Reece et al., 1994[22]	umbilical			no correlation
Ishimatsu et al., 1991[23]	umbilical		increased	no correlation
Johnstone et al., 1992[24]	umbilical			no correlation
Zimmermann et al., 1992[25]	umbilical	normal	normal	no correlation
Kofinas et al., 1991[29]	umbilical			no correlation
Salvesen et al., 1993[30]	umbilical	normal	normal	no correlation
Kofinas et al., 1991[29]	uterine			no correlation
Salvesen et al., 1993[30]	uterine	normal	normal	no correlation
Zimmermann et al., 1994[26]	uterine	normal	normal	no correlation

mellitus and reported increased impedance in those cases where histological examination of the decidual arteries after delivery showed severe vasculopathy[28]. The study confirmed a relationship between arcuate artery Doppler indices and downstream decidual vascular pathology. Kofinas et al. examined 31 pregnant women with gestational diabetes and 34 with insulin-dependent diabetes mellitus. Impedance to flow in the umbilical and uterine arteries during the third trimester was not different between patients with good glycemic control and those with poor control[29]. In contrast, impedance was significantly higher in patients with pre-eclampsia than in those without pre-eclampsia, regardless of glycemic control. It was concluded that Doppler investigation may be clinically useful only in diabetic pregnancies complicated by pre-eclampsia.

DOPPLER STUDIES OF THE FETAL MIDDLE CEREBRAL ARTERY AND AORTA

Diabetes mellitus is associated with an increased risk of fetal death, and data from cordocentesis have demonstrated an association between maternal hyperglycemia and fetal acidemia. The aim of Doppler ultrasound studies of the fetal middle cerebral artery and aorta is to examine whether the compromised fetus of a diabetic pregnancy demonstrates the same features of circulatory redistribution as seen in fetal hypoxemia due to uteroplacental insufficiency.

Salvesen *et al.* carried out a longitudinal Doppler study in 48 relatively well-controlled diabetic pregnancies[30]. With the exception of three pregnancies complicated by pre-eclampsia and/or intrauterine growth restriction, the uteroplacental and fetoplacental circulations were essentially normal. Thus, impedance to flow in the uterine and umbilical arteries and the PI or mean velocity in the middle cerebral artery or descending thoracic aorta were not significantly different from normal. It is of particular interest that normal Doppler results in the uterine and umbilical arteries and the fetal middle cerebral artery and aorta were also observed in five of six patients with diabetic nephropathy[31]. In all cases, iatrogenic delivery was carried out at 27–36 weeks because of worsening maternal proteinuric hypertension. Cordocentesis, performed within 24 hours before delivery, demonstrated these fetuses to be hypoxemic and acidemic. It was concluded that fetal acidemia in pregnancies complicated by diabetic nephropathy is not a consequence of impaired placental perfusion, and the degree of metabolic derangement may be obscured by the apparent normal growth of these fetuses and their failure to demonstrate blood flow redistribution. Another conclusion from this study is that uterine artery Doppler may be useful in distinguishing true pre-eclampsia (increased PI) from renal proteinuria and hypertension (normal PI).

Ishimatsu *et al.* measured impedance to flow in the fetal middle cerebral artery in 43 pregnant women with well-controlled diabetes mellitus at 24–38 weeks of gestation[32]. The PI was within the normal range and was not significantly associated with maternal serum glucose, fructosamine or glycosylated hemoglobin level. Reece *et al.* examined 30 pregnant women with insulin-dependent diabetes mellitus at 2-week intervals between 18 and 38 weeks of gestation[33]. They found no significant association between impedance to flow in the fetal aorta and fetal outcome. They concluded that fetal aortic Doppler velocimetry cannot be used as a means of assessing impending fetal compromise in offspring of diabetic mothers.

DOPPLER STUDIES OF THE FETAL HEART

Infants of diabetic mothers are at increased risk of hypertrophic cardiomyopathy. This disease is characterized by a thickening of the interventricular septum and ventricular walls and by systolic and diastolic dysfunction, which may result in congestive heart failure.

Rizzo *et al.* examined 40 well-controlled insulin-dependent diabetic pregnancies at 20–38 weeks of gestation and reported a significant increase in fetal interventricular septal thickness (Figure 1) and an associated decrease in the ratio between the peak velocities during early passive ventricular filling and active atrial filling at the level of the atrioventricular valves[34]. These findings, which were unrelated to maternal

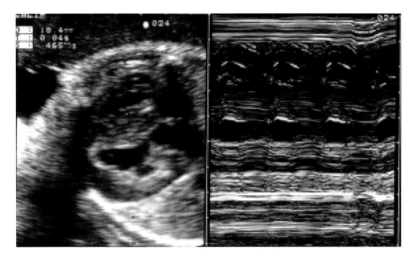

Figure 1 Real-time and M-mode tracing of a fetus of an insulin-dependent diabetic mother at 36 weeks of gestation. The interventricular wall septal thickness is increased (10 mm compared to the expected mean of 5 mm for this gestation)

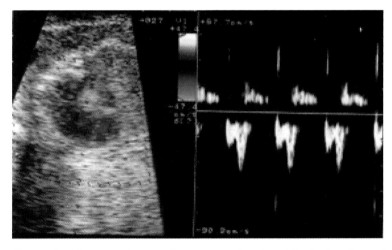

Figure 2 Flow velocity waveforms across the tricuspid valve in a fetus of an insulin-dependent diabetic mother at 32 weeks of gestation. The E/A ratio is decreased (0.48 compared to expected mean of 0.77 for this gestation)

glycosylated hemoglobin levels, suggest that, even in well-controlled maternal diabetes mellitus, there is fetal interventricular septal hypertrophy that affects cardiac diastolic function. A longitudinal study of 14 well-controlled, insulin-dependent diabetic pregnancies at 20–36 weeks of gestation confirmed the presence of hypertrophy in the interventricular septum and the right and left ventricular walls, as well as abnormal development of cardiac function – decrease in the ratio between early and active ventricular filling at the level of both the mitral and tricuspid valves (Figure 2)[35]. The cardiomegaly and cardiac dysfuncion increased with gestation but they were evident from as early as 20 weeks. Since the diabetic control in these pregnancies was good, it was suggested that fetal cardiomegaly may be the consequence of increased insulin sensitivity of the fetal myocardium. This hypothesis is supported by the data of Thorsson and Hintz, showing a reduction from fetus to adult in the number and affinity of insulin receptors[36].

The lower ratio between early and active ventricular filling at the level of the atrioventricular valves in fetuses of diabetic mothers may be due to impaired development of ventricular compliance, possibly secondary to cardiac wall thickening. In addition, the ratio may be influenced by reduced preload, as a consequence of the polycythemia, and therefore increased blood viscosity in fetuses of diabetic mothers. Thus, in a Doppler study of 37 fetuses of insulin-dependent diabetic mothers, immediately before an elective Cesarean section, the ratio between early and active ventricular filling was significantly and independently affected by both the interventricular wall thickness and fetal hematocrit[37].

Weber et al. performed serial evaluations of cardiac growth and ventricular diastolic filling using M-mode and Doppler echocardiography at 20–40 weeks of gestation and at 48–72 hours after birth in 11 fetuses of non-diabetic mothers and nine fetuses of well-controlled insulin-dependent diabetic mothers. Cardiac growth and birth weight in the two groups were similar[38]. Ventricular diastolic filling increased with gestation in both groups but the increase was delayed in the diabetic group. Tsyvian et al. examined 15 third-trimester pregnancies complicated by insulin-dependent maternal diabetes mellitus and reported a delay in fetal left ventricular filling, which may reflect changes in myocardial relaxation[39]. Weiner et al. examined 31 well-controlled insulin-dependent diabetic pregnancies at 22–40 weeks of gestation and reported that, after 34 weeks, in the fetuses of diabetic pregnancies, compared to normal pregnancies, there was a lower ratio between the peak velocities during early passive ventricular filling and active atrial filling at the level of the atrioventricular valves[40].

Macklon et al. examined well-controlled diabetic pregnancies at 18–20 weeks of gestation and reported that the fetal intraventricular septal thickness was increased, but transvalvular peak flow velocities and the duration of ventricular ejection in the fetal heart were not significantly different from normal[41]. It was concluded that, in fetuses of well-controlled diabetic pregnancies, altered cardiac morphology is evident early in pregnancy, before any obvious alteration in cardiac function. Rizzo *et al.* examined 27 insulin-dependent diabetic pregnancies from 12 weeks of gestation[42]. In the fetuses of diabetic mothers, compared to normal pregnancies, there was a lower ratio between early and active ventricular filling at the level of the atrioventricular valves, a higher percentage of reverse flow during atrial contraction in the inferior vena cava, and a higher proportion of cases with pulsations in the umbilical vein. These findings, demonstrating impaired development of cardiac and venous blood flow patterns from as early as at 12 weeks of gestation, were more evident in pregnancies with poorer glycemic control but they were also found in the presence of good metabolic control.

Peak velocities at the level of the aortic and pulmonary outflow tracts were significantly higher in fetuses of diabetic mothers than in normal fetuses[34]. The most likely explanations for the increased peak velocities are increased cardiac contractility (also found in postnatal studies in infants of diabetic mothers) and increased intracardiac flow volume due to the relatively large size of such fetuses, since cardiac output is a function of fetal weight. These abnormalities in cardiac hemodynamics also impair the venous circulation. Rizzo *et al.* carried out a cross-sectional study of 62 third-trimester fetuses in insulin-dependent diabetic pregnancies and reported that increased preload index in the inferior vena cava (in the absence of alterations in fetal peripheral vessels) was associated with a lower umbilical arterial blood pH and higher hematocrit at birth, as well as increased neonatal morbidity[43]. These findings suggest that the mechanisms inducing fetal distress in diabetic pregnancies (where the development of hypertrophic cardiomyopathy plays a pivotal role in the genesis of fetal distress) are different from those in fetuses with intrauterine growth restriction, where the change in cardiac function is secondary to the alteration in peripheral resistance.

In neonates from normal pregnancies, the ratio between early and active ventricular filling at the level of the atrioventricular valves increases during the first few days of postnatal life; the early wave is usually higher than the active one, resulting in a ratio between early and active ventricular filling that is higher than one. In newborns of diabetic mothers, there are no changes in this ratio during the first 5 days of life and its value remains lower than one[44]. These anomalies might explain the relatively high incidence of transitory tachypnea and pulmonary edema in neonates from diabetic pregnancies. The cardiac hypertrophy of fetuses of diabetic mothers resolves during the first year of postnatal life. However, it is possible that the cardiac hypertrophy and dysfunction observed in intrauterine life may affect cardiac function in adult life.

CONCLUSIONS

- In maternal diabetes mellitus, impedance to flow in the uterine and umbilical arteries is not related to either short-term or long-term maternal glycemic control.

- In maternal diabetes mellitus, impedance to flow in the uterine arteries is normal, even in patients with nephropathy and vasculopathy. However, increased impedance, as in non–diabetic pregnancies, identifies a group at high risk for subsequent development of pre-eclampsia and/or intrauterine growth restriction.

- In maternal diabetes mellitus, increased impedance to flow in the umbilical artery is associated with the development of pre-eclampsia and/or intrauterine growth restriction. There is contradictory evidence concerning a possible increase in impedance in pregnancies with maternal vasculopathy.

- In maternal diabetes mellitus, there is no evidence of redistribution in the fetal circulation with decreased PI in the middle cerebral artery and increased PI in the descending thoracic aorta. This is presumably because, in diabetes, there may be acute fluctuations in fetal blood pH, since the latter is associated with the maternal glucose concentration. Furthermore, unlike intrauterine growth restriction, in diabetes metabolic derangements in the fetus may lead to acidemia without hypoxemia. Therefore, the classic redistribution seen in fetal hypoxemia due to uteroplacental insufficiency may not occur even in severely compromised fetuses, and it is therefore important not to be misled by apparently normal fetal Doppler results.

- In maternal diabetes mellitus, the fetus is at increased risk of hypertrophic cardiomyopathy. This disease is characterized by a thickening of the interventricular septum and cardiac dysfunction, which may be evident from as early as 12 weeks of gestation.

REFERENCES

1. Economides DL, Nicolaides KH. Blood glucose and oxygen tension in small for gestational age fetuses. *Am J Obstet Gynecol* 1989;160:385–9

2. Salvesen DR, Brudenell JM, Proudler A, Crook D, Nicolaides KH. Fetal pancreatic β-cell function in pregnancies complicated by maternal diabetes mellitus. *Am J Obstet Gynecol* 1993;168:1363–9

3. Pedersen J. *The Pregnant Diabetic and Her Newborn*, 2nd edn. Baltimore: Williams and Wilkins, 1977:211–20

4. Wang HS, Chard T. The role of insulin-like growth factor-I and insulin-like growth factor-binding protein-1 in the control of human fetal growth. *J Endocrinol* 1992;132:11–19

5. Bradley RJ, Brudenell JM, Nicolaides KH. Fetal acidosis and hyperlacticaemia diagnosed by cordocentesis in pregnancies complicated by maternal diabetes mellitus. *Diabet Med* 1991;8:464–8

6. Salvesen DR, Brudenell JM, Nicolaides KH. Fetal polycythemia and thrombocytopenia in pregnancies complicated by maternal diabetes mellitus. *Am J Obstet Gynecol* 1992;166:1287–92

7. Salvesen DR, Brudenell JM, Nicolaides KH. Fetal plasma erythropoietin in pregnancies complicated by maternal diabetes. *Am J Obstet Gynecol* 1993;168:88–94

8. Robillard JE, Sessions C, Kennedy RL, Smith FG. Metabolic effect of constant hypertonic glucose infusion in well oxygenated fetuses. *Am J Obstet Gynecol* 1978;130:199–203

9. Phillips AF, Dubin JW, Matty PJ, Raye JR. Arterial hypoxemia and hyperinsulinemia in the chronically hyperglycemic fetal lamb. *Pediatr Res* 1982;16:653–8

10. Phillips AF, Porte PJ, Stabinsky S, Rosenkrantz TS, Raye JR. Effects of chronic fetal hyperglycemia upon oxygen consumption in the ovine uterus and conceptus. *J Clin Invest* 1984;74:279–86

11. Phillips AF, Rosenkrantz TS, Porte PJ, Raye JR. The effect of chronic fetal hyperglycemia on substrate uptake by the ovine fetus and conceptus. *Pediatr Res* 1985;19:659–66

12. Hay WW, DiGiacomo JE, Meznarich HK, Zerbe G. Effects of glucose and insulin on fetal glucose oxidation and oxygen consumption. *Am J Physiol* 1989;256:E704–13

13. Shelly HJ, Bassett JM, Milner RDG. Control of carbohydrate metabolism in the fetus and newborn. *Br Med Bull* 1975;31:37–43

14. Fox H. Pathology of the placenta in maternal diabetes mellitus. *Obstet Gynecol* 1969;34:792–8

15. Olofsson P, Lingman G, Marsal K, Sjoberg NO. Fetal blood flow in diabetic pregnancy. *J Perinat Med* 1987;15:545–53

16. Ursem NT, Clark EB, Keller BB, Wladimiroff JW. Fetal heart rate and umbilical artery velocity variability in pregnancies complicated by insulin-dependent diabetes mellitus. *Ultrasound Obstet Gynecol* 1999;13:312–16

17. Bracero L, Schulman H, Fleischer A, Farmakides G, Rochelson B. Umbilical artery velocimetry in diabetes and pregnancy. *Obstet Gynecol* 1986;68:654–8

18. Bracero LA, Figueroa R, Byrne DW, Han HJ. Comparison of umbilical Doppler velocimetry, nonstress testing, and biophysical profile in pregnancies complicated by diabetes. *J Ultrasound Med* 1996;15:301–8

19. Bracero LA, Evanco J, Byrne DW. Doppler velocimetry discordancy of the uterine arteries in pregnancies complicated by diabetes. *J Ultrasound Med* 1997;16:387–93

20. Landon MB, Gabbe SG, Bruner JP, Ludmir J. Doppler umbilical artery velocimetry in pregnancy complicated by insulin-dependent diabetes mellitus. *Obstet Gynecol* 1989;73:961–5

21. Dicker D, Goldman JA, Yeshaya A, Peleg D. Umbilical artery velocimetry in insulin dependent diabetes mellitus (IDDM) pregnancies. *J Perinat Med* 1990;18:391–5

22. Reece EA, Hagay Z, Assimakopoulos E, Moroder W, Gabrielli S, DeGennaro N, Homko C, O'Connor T, Wiznitzer A. Diabetes mellitus in pregnancy and the assessment of umbilical artery waveforms using pulsed Doppler ultrasonography. *J Ultrasound Med* 1994;13:73–80

23. Ishimatsu J, Yoshimura O, Manabe A, Hotta M, Matsunaga T, Matsuzaki T, Tetsuou M, Hamada T. Umbilical artery blood flow velocity waveforms in pregnancy complicated by diabetes mellitus. *Arch Gynecol Obstet* 1991;248:123–7

24. Johnstone FD, Steel JM, Haddad NG, Hoskins PR, Greer IA, Chambers S. Doppler umbilical artery flow velocity waveforms in diabetic pregnancy. *Br J Obstet Gynaecol* 1992;99:135–40

25. Zimmermann P, Kujansuu E, Tuimala R. Doppler velocimetry of the umbilical artery in pregnancies complicated by insulin-dependent diabetes mellitus. *Eur J Obstet Gynecol Reprod Biol* 1992;47: 85–93

26. Zimmermann P, Kujansuu E, Tuimala R. Doppler flow velocimetry of the uterine and uteroplacental circulation in pregnancies complicated by insulin-dependent diabetes mellitus. *J Perinat Med* 1994;22:137–47

27. Haddad B, Uzan M, Tchobroutsky C, Uzan S, Papiernik-Berkhauer E. Predictive value of uterine Doppler waveform during pregnancies complicated by diabetes. *Fetal Diagn Ther* 1993;8:119–25

28. Barth WH Jr, Genest DR, Riley LE, Frigoletto FD Jr, Benacerraf BR, Greene MF. Uterine arcuate artery Doppler and decidual microvascular pathology in pregnancies complicated by type I diabetes mellitus. *Ultrasound Obstet Gynecol* 1996;8:98–103

29. Kofinas AD, Penry M, Swain M. Uteroplacental Doppler flow velocity waveform analysis correlates poorly with glycemic control in diabetic pregnant women. *Am J Perinatol* 1991;8:273–7

30. Salvesen DR, Higueras MT, Mansur CA, Freeman J, Brudenell JM, Nicolaides KH. Placental and fetal Doppler velocimetry in pregnancies complicated by maternal diabetes mellitus. *Am J Obstet Gynecol* 1993;168:645–52

31. Salvesen DR, Higueras MT, Brudenell JM, Drury PL, Nicolaides KH. Doppler velocimetry and fetal heart rate studies in nephropathic diabetics. *Am J Obstet Gynecol* 1992;167:1297–303

32. Ishimatsu J, Matsuzaki T, Yakushiji M, Hamada T. Blood flow velocity waveforms of the fetal middle cerebral artery in pregnancies complicated by diabetes mellitus. *Kurume Med J* 1995;42: 161–6

33. Reece EA, Hagay Z, Moroder W, DeGennaro N, Homko C, Wiznitzer A. Is there a correlation between aortic Doppler velocimetric findings in diabetic pregnant women and fetal outcome? *J Ultrasound Med* 1996;15:437–40

34. Rizzo G, Arduini D, Romanini C. Cardiac function in fetuses of type I diabetic mothers. *Am J Obstet Gynecol* 1991;164:837–43

35. Rizzo G, Arduini D, Romanini C. Accelerated cardiac growth and abnormal cardiac flow in fetuses of type I diabetic mothers. *Obstet Gynecol* 1992;80:369–76

36. Thorsson AV, Hintz RL. Insulin receptors in the newborn: Increase in receptor affinity and number. *N Engl J Med* 1977:297;908–12

37. Rizzo G, Pietropolli A, Capponi A, Cacciatore C, Arduini D, Romanini C. Analysis of factors influencing ventricular filling patterns in fetuses of type I diabetic mothers. *J Perinat Med* 1994;22:149–57

38. Weber HS, Botti JJ, Baylen BG. Sequential longitudinal evaluation of cardiac growth and ventricular diastolic filling in fetuses of well controlled diabetic mothers. *Pediatr Cardiol* 1994;15:184–9

39. Tsyvian P, Malkin K, Artemieva O, Wladimiroff JW. Assessment of left ventricular filling in normally grown fetuses, growth-restricted fetuses and fetuses of diabetic mothers. *Ultrasound Obstet Gynecol* 1998;12:33–8

40. Weiner Z, Zloczower M, Lerner A, Zimmer E, Itskovitz-Eldor J. Cardiac compliance in fetuses of diabetic women. *Obstet Gynecol* 1999;93:948–51

41. Macklon NS, Hop WC, Wladimiroff JW. Fetal cardiac function and septal thickness in diabetic pregnancy: a controlled observational and reproducibility study. *Br J Obstet Gynaecol* 1998;105: 661–6

42. Rizzo G, Arduini D, Capponi A, Romanini C. Cardiac and venous blood flow in fetuses of insulin-dependent diabetic mothers: evidence of abnormal hemodynamics in early gestation. *Am J Obstet Gynecol* 1995;173:1775–81

43. Rizzo G, Capponi A, Angelini E, Mazzoleni A. Romanini C. Inferior cava velocity waveform predict neonatal complications in fetuses of insulin dependent diabetic mothers. In press

44. Mace S, Hirschfeld SS, Riggs T, Faranoff AA, Mecketz IR. Echocardiographic abnormalities in infants of diabetic mothers. *J Pediatr* 1979;95:1013–19

8

Doppler studies in preterm prelabor amniorrhexis

PATHOPHYSIOLOGY

Preterm delivery occurs in less than 10% of pregnancies but accounts for more than 70% of all neonatal deaths. Approximately one-third of preterm deliveries are associated with preterm prelabor amniorrhexis and, in a high proportion of such cases, the underlying cause may be ascending infection from the lower genital tract. Thus, positive amniotic fluid cultures, with organisms commonly found in the vagina, are present in about one-third of cases with preterm prelabor amniorrhexis and in one-third of these there is fetal bacteremia.

In a study of 69 pregnancies with preterm prelabor amniorrhexis, the diagnosis of intrauterine infection was based on the results of culture of amniotic fluid and fetal blood obtained by amniocentesis and cordocentesis, respectively[1]. In patients with fetal bacteremia, there was spontaneous delivery within 5 days of amniorrhexis, whereas, in those with negative fetal blood and amniotic fluid cultures, the interval between amniorrhexis and delivery was prolonged by up to 5 months and subsequent cultures of blood obtained from the umbilical cord at delivery or from the neonates were negative[1]. These findings suggest that, first, infection is one of the causes rather than the consequence of amniorrhexis, and, second, in preterm prelabor amniorrhexis, infection may be the cause of subsequent preterm labor and delivery. The likely mechanism for the link between infection and labor is infection-mediated release of cytokines which stimulate the production of prostaglandins that induce uterine contractions[2,3].

In pregnancies complicated by preterm prelabor amniorrhexis, there are essentially two causes of perinatal death: prematurity and pulmonary hypoplasia. In cases with intrauterine infection, delivery occurs within a few days and therefore survival depends on the gestation at amniorrhexis[1]. Postnatal survival increases from less than 10% before

24 weeks to more than 90% by 30 weeks. In those patients with no infection, pregnancy may be prolonged by several weeks and, in these cases, there is a risk of postnatal death due to pulmonary hypoplasia[4]. The risk of death is inversely related to the gestation at amniorrhexis and decreases from approximately 50% for those with amniorrhexis before 20 weeks, to 20% for those with amniorrhexis at 20–24 weeks and to less than 5% for amniorrhexis after 24 weeks. Consequently, in the management of pregnancies complicated by amniorrhexis, the major issue is prediction of intrauterine infection and pulmonary hypoplasia.

Fetal blood gases

Cordocentesis in pregnancies with preterm prelabor amniorrhexis has demonstrated that the mean umbilical venous blood pO_2 and pH are not significantly different from the appropriate normal mean for gestation, and there are no significant differences between those with positive or negative fetal blood and amniotic fluid cultures[5]. These findings suggest that, in the presence of intrauterine infection, fetal oxygenation is not impaired.

DOPPLER STUDIES

Prediction of intrauterine infection

The rationale for the use of Doppler in pregnancies with preterm prelabor amniorrhexis is that infection of the amniotic fluid and choriodecidua causes constriction of the umbilical cord and chorionic vessels and may consequently impair fetal perfusion[6-12].

Doppler studies of the umbilical arterial circulation in pregnancies with chorioamnionitis have provided conflicting results, with some reporting an increase and others no change in impedance to flow. Thus, in two cross-sectional studies, involving a total of 35 patients with clinical chorioamnionitis, impedance to flow in the umbilical arteries was always normal[13,14]. In a longitudinal study of 22 patients with preterm prelabor amniorrhexis and umbilical vasculitis, although there was an increase of impedance in the umbilical arteries 24 hours before delivery compared to previous measurements, impedance had remained within the normal range[15]. In another longitudinal study of uterine and umbilical arteries in 60 patients with amniorrhexis, including 12 who developed clinical chorioamnionitis, there was no significant increase in impedance, even in measurements taken within 24 hours before delivery[16].

Carroll *et al.* performed Doppler studies immediately before cordocentesis and amniocentesis for bacteriological studies in 69 pregnancies with preterm prelabor amniorrhexis[5]. The mean pulsatility indices in the uterine and umbilical arteries and in the fetal middle cerebral arteries and thoracic aorta were not significantly different from the appropriate normal mean for gestation and there were no significant differences in these values between those with and without intrauterine infection[5].

These findings suggest that chorioamnionitis is not associated with a major degree of vasoconstriction in the uteroplacental or fetoplacental circulation. Consequently, Doppler does not provide a clinically useful distinction between infected and non-infected cases. However, Doppler studies in pregnancies with suspected amniorrhexis may be useful in the differential diagnosis from oligohydramnios due to uteroplacental insufficiency and intrauterine growth restriction. In the latter, there is an increase in impedance to flow in the uterine and/or umbilical arteries with decreased pulsatility index in the fetal cerebral vessels and increased pulsatility index (PI) in the descending thoracic aorta (see Chapter 4).

Prediction of pulmonary hypoplasia

Amniorrhexis before 25 weeks of gestation is associated with the development of pulmonary hypoplasia and hypertension. Suggested mechanisms for the development of pulmonary hypoplasia include:

(1) Extrinsic compression of the fetal lungs, which interferes with normal development;

(2) Excessive loss of lung fluid, either due to extrinsic compression of the fetal thorax or decrease in intra-amniotic pressure and increase in the alveolar–amniotic pressure gradient[17]; and

(3) Cessation of fetal breathing movements, because, in animal studies, transection of the cervical spinal cord and consequent interruption of breathing movements result in pulmonary hypoplasia[18].

Attempts at antenatal prediction of pulmonary hypoplasia in pregnancies with preterm prelabor amniorrhexis have focused on ultrasonographic assessment of lung size, amniotic fluid volume and fetal breathing movements[19]. Studies examining fetal thoracic circumference and lung size have reported favorable results in the prediction of pulmonary hypoplasia[20,21], whereas studies that attempted to quantify the degree of oligohydramnios or fetal breathing movements have generally reported poor prediction[19–23].

Prediction of pulmonary hypoplasia has also been attempted by antenatal Doppler studies[24]. Blood flow in the ductus arteriosus, as assessed by Doppler ultrasound, is altered by breathing movements. In a study of 12 cases of preterm prelabor amniorrhexis and severe oligohydramnios, the alteration in ductal blood flow by breathing movements was normal in seven cases with normal lungs, and reduced in all five cases with pulmonary hypoplasia[25]. Doppler studies in fetuses with pulmonary hypoplasia, due to multicystic kidneys or obstructive uropathy, reported increased impedance to flow in the branches of the pulmonary artery, consistent with high peripheral pulmonary vascular resistance[26–29].

Rizzo *et al.* meaured the PI in the peripheral pulmonary arteries in 20 pregnancies complicated by amniorrhexis before 24 weeks of gestation[30]. In fetuses that subsequently developed pulmonary hypoplasia, the PI was increased from as early as 2 weeks after amniorrhexis (Figure 1). The PI in the peripheral pulmonary arteries was above the 95th centile of the normal range in 62.5% of those that developed pulmonary hypoplasia[30].

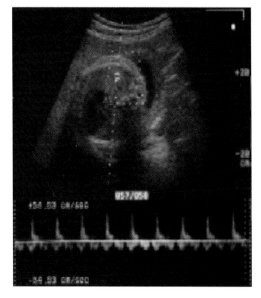
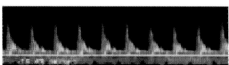

Figure 1 Flow velocity waveforms (left) from the fetal peripheral pulmonary artery at 26 weeks of gestation in a pregnancy complicated by ruptured membranes and subsequent neonatal death due to pulmonary hypoplasia. The waveform (right) was from a pregnancy not resulting in pulmonary hypoplasia

CONCLUSIONS

- Preterm prelabor amniorrhexis is associated with a high risk of preterm delivery, due to intrauterine infection, as well as neonatal death, due to pulmonary hypoplasia.

- In pregnancies with preterm prelabor amniorrhexis, intrauterine infection is not associated with altered fetal oxygenation or a major degree of vasoconstriction in the uteroplacental or fetoplacental circulation.

- In pregnancies with preterm prelabor amniorrhexis, Doppler assessment does not provide a clinically useful distinction between infected and non-infected cases. The pulsatility indices in the uterine and umbilical arteries and in the fetal middle cerebral arteries and thoracic aorta are not significantly different from normal and there are no significant differences between these values in those with and without intrauterine infection.

- In pregnancies with preterm prelabor amniorrhexis, Doppler assessment may be useful in the prediction of pulmonary hypoplasia. Thus, in fetuses that subsequently develop pulmonary hypoplasia, impedance in the peripheral pulmonary arteries is increased from as early as 2 weeks after amniorrhexis.

REFERENCES

1. Carroll SG, Ville Y, Greenough A, Gamsu H, Patel B, Philpott-Howard J, Nicolaides KH. Preterm prelabour amniorrhexis: intrauterine infection and interval between membrane rupture and delivery. *Arch Dis Child* 1995;72:F43–6

2. Gomez R, Romero R, Mazor M, Ghezzi F, David C, Yoon BH. The role of infection in preterm labour and delivery. In Elder MG, Lamont RF, Romero R, eds. *Preterm Labour.* Edinburgh: Churchill Livingstone, 1997:85

3. Carroll SG, Abbas A, Ville Y, Meher-Homjii H, Nicolaides KH. Concentration of fetal plasma and amniotic fluid interleukin-1 in pregnancies complicated by preterm prelabour amniorrhexis. *J Clin Pathol* 1995;48:368–71

4. Carroll SG, Blott M, Nicolaides KH. Preterm prelabor amniorrhexis: outcome of livebirths. *Obstet Gynecol* 1995;86:18–25

5. Carroll SG, Papaioannou S, Nicolaides KH. Doppler studies of the placental and fetal circulation in pregnancies with preterm prelabour amniorrhexis. *Ultrasound Obstet Gynecol* 1995;5:184–8

6. Howard RB, Hosokawa T, Maguire MH. Pressor and depressor actions of prostanoids in the intact human feto-placental vascular bed. *Prostaglandins Leukotrienes Med* 1986;21:323–30

7. Mak KK-W, Gude NM, Walters WAW, Boura ALA. Effects of vasoactive autocoids on the human umbilical-fetal placental vasculature. *Br J Obstet Gynaecol* 1984;91:99–106

8. Altura BM, Malaviya AD, Reich CF, Orkin LR. Effects of vasoactive agents on isolated human umbilical arteries and veins. *Am J Physiol* 1972;222:345–55

9. Hyde S, Smotherman J, Moore J, Altshulter G. A model of bacterially induced umbilical vein spasm, relevant to fetal hypoperfusion. *Obstet Gynecol* 1989;73:966–70

10. Hellerqvist CG, Rojas J, Green RS, Sell S, Sundell H, Stahlman MT. Studies of group B, beta-hemolytic streptococcus. Isolation and partial characterization of an extracellular toxin. *Pediatr Res* 1981;15:892–8

11. Sandberg K, Englehardt B, Hellerqvist C, Sundell H. Pulmonary response to group B streptococcal toxin in young lambs. *J Appl Physiol* 1987;63:2024–30

12. Bjoro K, Stray-Pedersen. Effects of vasoactive autocoids on different segments of human umbilico-placental vessels. *Gynecol Obstet Invest* 1986;22:1–6

13. Brar HS, Medearis AL, Platt LD. Relationship of systolic/diastolic ratios from umbilical velocimetry to fetal heart rate. *Am J Obstet Gynecol* 1989;160:188–91

14. Leo MV, Skurnick JH, Ganesh VV, Adhate A, Apuzzio JJ. Clinical chorioamnionitis is not predicted by umbilical artery doppler velocimetry in patients with premature rupture of membranes. *Obstet Gynecol* 1992;79:916–8

15. Fleming AD, Salafia CM, Vintzileos AM, Rodis JF, Campbell WA, Bantham F. The relationships among umbilical artery velocimetry, fetal biophysical profile, and placental inflammation in preterm premature rupture of the membranes. *Am J Obstet Gynecol* 1991;164:38–41

16. Abramowicz JS, Sherer DM, Warsof SL, Levy DL. Fetoplacental and uteroplacental Doppler blood flow velocity analysis in premature rupture of membranes. *Am J Perinatol* 1992;9:353–6

17. Nicolini U, Fisk NM, Rodeck CH, Talbert DG, Wigglesworth JS. Low amniotic pressure in oligohydramnios – is this the cause of pulmonary hypoplasia? *Am J Obstet Gynecol* 1989;161:1098–101

18. Wigglesworth JS, Desai R. Effects on lung growth of cervical cord section in the rabbit fetus. *Early Hum Dev* 1979;3:51–65

19. Carroll SG, Papaioannou S, Nicolaides KH. Assessment of fetal activity and amniotic fluid volume in the prediction of intrauterine infection in preterm prelabor amniorrhexis. *Am J Obstet Gynecol* 1995;172:1427–35

20. Blott M, Greenough A, Nicolaides KH, Campbell S. The ultrasonographic assessment of the fetal thorax and fetal breathing movements in the prediction of pulmonary hypoplasia. *Early Hum Dev* 1990;21:143–51

21. Roberts AB, Mitchell JM. Direct ultrasonographic measurement of fetal lung length in normal pregnancies and pregnancies complicated by prolonged rupture of membranes. *Am J Obstet Gynecol* 1990;163:1560–6

22. Rotschild A, Ling EW, Puterman ML, Farquharson D. Neonatal outcome after prolonged preterm rupture of the membranes. *Am J Obstet Gynecol* 1990;162:46–52

23. Moessinger AC, Higgins A, Fox HE, Rey HR. Fetal breathing movements are not a reliable predictor of continued lung development in pregnancies complicated by oligohydramnios. *Lancet* 1987;ii:1297–9

24. Wladimiroff JW. Predicting pulmonary hypoplasia: assessment of lung volume or lung function or both? *Ultrasound Obstet Gynecol* 1998;11:164–6

25. Van Eyck J, van der Mooren K, Wladimiroff JW. Ductus arteriosus flow velocity modulation by fetal breathing movements as a measure of fetal lung development. *Am J Obstet Gynecol* 1990;163: 558–66

26. Laudy JA, Gaillard JL, v d Anker JN, Tibboel D, Wladimiroff JW. Doppler ultrasound imaging: a new technique to detect lung hypoplasia before birth? *Ultrasound Obstet Gynecol* 1996;7:189–92

27. Mitchell JM, Roberts AB, Lee A. Doppler waveforms from the pulmonary arterial system in normal fetuses and those with pulmonary hypoplasia. *Ultrasound Obstet Gynecol* 1998;11:167–72

28. Oshimura S, Masuzaki H, Miura K, Muta K, Gotoh H, Ishimaru T Diagnosis of fetal pulmonary hypoplasia by measurement of blood flow velocity waveforms of pulmonary arteries with Doppler ultrasonography. *Am J Obstet Gynecol* 1999;180:441–6

29. Chaoui R, Kalache K., Tennestedt C, Lenz F, Vogel M. Pulmonary arterial Doppler velocimetry in fetuses with lung hypoplasia. *Eur J Obstet Gynecol Reprod Biol* 1999;84:179–185

30. Rizzo G, Capponi A., Angelini E, Mazzoleni A, Romanini C. Blood flow velocity waveforms from fetal peripheral pulmonary arteries in pregnancies with preterm premature rupture of membranes: relationship with pulmonary hypoplasia. *Ultrasound Obstet Gynecol* 2000;in press

9

Doppler studies in maternal autoimmune disease

SYSTEMIC LUPUS ERYTHEMATOSUS

Systemic lupus erythematosus, which affects about one in 1000 adults, is an idiopathic multisystem chronic inflammatory disease, characterized by the presence of circulating autoantibodies directed against nuclear antigens.

In pregnant women with systemic lupus erythematosus, the rate of fetal loss in the first trimester is similar to that in normal women (about 15%), but, in the second and third trimesters, the fetal loss rate is about 10%[1,2]. The mechanism for this increase in fetal loss is unclear but may be related to placental dysfunction. The most sensitive predictor of fetal death is the presence of antiphospholipid antibodies[3–5].

About 25% of pregnancies in women with systemic lupus erythematosus are complicated by pre-eclampsia[3]. The reason for this increased frequency of pre-eclampsia may be related to the underlying renal disease[6]. Fetal growth restriction is found in about 20% of pregnancies[1]. Distinguishing between an exacerbation of systemic lupus erythematosus involving active nephritis and pre-eclampsia is difficult, since they may both present with proteinuria, hypertension and evidence of multi-organ dysfunction. In the typical problem case, the patient develops hypertension and increasing proteinuria in the latter half of pregnancy. Elevated levels of anti-dsDNA and an active urinary sediment strongly suggest lupus. In severe and confusing cases, renal biopsy may be necessary to make the correct diagnosis.

Neonatal lupus erythematosus, with a birth prevalence of about one in 20 000, is characterized by dermatological, cardiac or hematological abnormalities. The condition is due to maternal autoantibodies, particularly anti-Ro/SS-A and anti-SS-B/La, that cross the placenta[7]. About half of the mothers who deliver an infant with neonatal lupus erythematosus have systemic lupus erythematosus or another autoimmune disease. The risk of a mother with anti-SS-A/Ro and/or anti-SS-B/La having a fetus or neonate with neonatal lupus erythematosus is fairly low and among all mothers with systemic lupus erythematosus, the risk of neonatal lupus erythematosus is less than 5%[8]. The cardiac lesions associated with the condition are congenital complete heart block and endocardial fibroelastosis. The usual presentation is a fixed fetal bradycardia of 60–80 beats per min presenting at 15–25 weeks of gestation; in some cases there is associated hydrops fetalis. The histological lesion is one of fibrosis and interruption of the conduction system, especially in the area of the atrioventricular node. Because the lesion is permanent, a pacemaker may be necessary for neonatal survival. After prenatal diagnosis of fetal heart block, administration of a glucocorticoid to the mother is associated with improvement in fetal cardiac function and limitation of further immunological damage to the fetal heart[9,10].

ANTIPHOSPHOLIPID SYNDROME

Antiphospholipid syndrome is an autoimmune condition characterized by the production of moderate to high levels of antiphospholipid antibodies (lupus anticoagulant or anticardiolipin antibody) and at least one clinical feature (venous or arterial thrombosis, autoimmune thrombocytopenia and/or pregnancy loss). The risk of thrombosis in pregnancy in women with antiphospholipid syndrome is sufficiently substantial to warrant prophylactic treatment with heparin.

Antiphospholipid syndrome is associated with early pregnancy loss; antiphospholipid antibodies are found in about 10% of women with recurrent first-trimester pregnancy loss (compared to about 2.5% in controls)[11–15]. About 50% of women with antiphospholipid syndrome develop pre-eclampsia, which may start from as early as 15 weeks, or worsening hypertension[16,17] and about 10% of women with severe early-onset (before 34 weeks) pre-eclampsia have antiphospholipid antibodies. The rate of pre-eclampsia does not appear to be markedly diminished by treatment with either glucocorticoids with low-dose aspirin or heparin with low-dose aspirin. The syndrome is also associated with fetal growth impairment, which is found in about 30% of treated pregnancies[16,17]. In women with antiphospholipid syndrome, treatment with thromboprophylactic doses of heparin and low-dose aspirin improves the chances of a successful pregnancy outcome[18–21].

DOPPLER STUDIES

In pregnancies complicated by maternal systemic lupus erythematosus, increased impedance to flow in the umbilical arteries is associated with increased risk of pre-eclampsia and intrauterine growth restriction. Thus, Kerslake *et al.* carried out serial Doppler studies in 56 pregnancies complicated by maternal systemic lupus erythematosus[22]. They reported that the absence of end-diastolic frequencies in the umbilical artery was a good predictor of the need for subsequent delivery by Cesarean section, whereas the presence of end-diastolic frequencies was associated with normotensive pregnancy[22]. Similarly, Farine *et al.* examined 56 pregnancies complicated by maternal systemic lupus erythematosus and reported that absent or reversed end-diastolic frequencies, which were detected in 11% of the patients, were associated with increased risk of pre-eclampsia and intrauterine growth restriction[23].

In systemic lupus erythematosus, it is uncertain if impedance to flow in the uterine arteries is increased. Thus, Weiner *et al.* carried out serial Doppler studies of the uterine and umbilical arteries in five patients with systemic lupus erythematosus from week 10 to term[24]. Impedance to flow in the uterine artery was within the normal range in all cases, whereas most values from the umbilical artery were above the 95th centile of the normal range. All five pregnancies resulted in healthy live births but one infant was growth-restricted; the highest impedance in the umbilical artery was observed in the case of growth restriction. Guzman *et al.* examined 27 pregnancies in women with systemic lupus erythematosus[25]. In 18 pregnancies, there was normal impedance in both the uterine and umbilical arteries and they all had normal outcomes. In five pregnancies, there was normal impedance in the uterine arteries but increased impedance in the umbilical artery and, in this group, there were two cases of intrauterine growth restriction. In four pregnancies, there was increased impedance in both vessels; in all four, there was intrauterine growth restriction and three resulted in intrauterine or neonatal death.

In antiphospholipid syndrome there is thrombosis of the uteroplacental vasculature and placental infarction. There is some evidence that, in pregnancies with antiphospholipid syndrome, increased impedance in the uterine arteries identifies those cases that subsequently develop pre-eclampsia and intrauterine growth restriction. Thus, Caruso *et al.* examined 28 pregnancies in women with antiphospholipid syndrome and reported that increased impedance in the uterine arteries at 18–24 weeks of gestation provided useful prediction of both pre-eclampsia and intrauterine growth restriction[26]. In this respect, the findings of Doppler studies in predicting the outcome of pregnancies with the antiphospholipid syndrome may be similar to those with placental insufficiency due to impaired trophoblastic invasion of the maternal spiral arteries. However, Trudinger *et al.* suggested that, in the antiphospholipid syndrome, infarction of the placental vessels may be an acute phenomenon causing rapid deterioration in the fetal condition without impairment in growth, which would necessitate chronic placental insufficiency[27]. They examined six pregnancies in women with antiphospholipid syndrome and reported increased impedance to flow in the umbilical artery in four of the cases, despite the absence of pre-eclampsia or intrauterine growth restriction. Further evidence emphasizing the difference in the implications of antiphospholipid syndrome from impaired trophoblastic invasion was provided by the studies of Carroll[28]. He examined 28 pregnancies complicated by antiphospholipid syndrome and reported that, in five of the six cases associated with intrauterine growth restriction, impedance to flow in the umbilical arteries was increased, whereas only two of these patients demonstrated abnormally elevated impedance in the uterine arteries.

CONCLUSIONS

- Systemic lupus erythematosus is associated with increased risk of pre-eclampsia, intrauterine growth restriction and perinatal death.

- In systemic lupus erythematosus, increased impedance to flow in the umbilical arteries is associated with increased risk of pre-eclampsia and intrauterine growth restriction.

- In systemic lupus erythematosus, it is uncertain if impedance to flow in the uterine arteries is increased.

- Antiphospholipid syndrome is characterized by thrombosis of the uteroplacental vasculature and placental infarction, and is associated with early pregnancy loss, pre-eclampsia and intrauterine growth restriction.

- In antiphospholipid syndrome, the development of pre-eclampsia and intrauterine growth restriction is preceded by increased impedance to flow in the umbilical arteries and possibly the uterine arteries.

REFERENCES

1. Mintz R, Niz J, Gutierrez G, Garcia-Alonso A, Karchmer S. Prospective study of pregnancy in systemic lupus erythematosus: results of a multidisciplinary approach. *J Rheumatol* 1986;13:732–9
2. Zulman JI, Talal N, Hoffman GS, Epstein WV. Problems associated with the management of pregnancies in patients with systemic lupus erythematosus. *J Rheumatol* 1979;7:37–49
3. Lockshin MD, Qamar T, Druzin ML. Hazards of lupus pregnancy. *J Rheumatol* 1987;14:214–17
4. Lockshin MD, Druzin ML, Goei S, *et al.* Antibody to cardiolipin as a predictor of fetal distress or death in pregnant patients with systemic lupus erythematosus. *N Engl J Med* 1985;313:152–6
5. Englert HJ, Derue GM, Loizou S, *et al.* Pregnancy and lupus: prognostic indicators and response to treatment. *Q J Med* 1988;66:125–36

6. Fisher KA, Luger A, Spargo BH, *et al.* Hypertension in pregnancy: clinical-pathologic correlations and remote prognosis. *Medicine* 1981;60:267–76

7. Buyon JP, Winchester RJ, Slade SG, *et al.* Identification of mothers at risk for congenital heart block and other neonatal lupus syndromes in their children: comparison of enzyme-linked immuno-sorbent assay and immunoblot for measurement of anti-SS-A/Ro and anti-SS-B/La antibodies. *Arthr Rheum* 1993;36:1263–73

8. Lockshin MD, Bonfa E, Elkon D, Druzin ML. Neonatal lupus risk to newborns of mothers with systemic lupus erythematosus. *Arthr Rheum* 1988;31:697–701

9. Rider LG, Buyon JP, Rutledge J, Sherry DD. Treatment of neonatal lupus: case and report and review of the literature. *J Rheumatol* 1993;20:1208

10. Copel JA, Buyon JP, Kleinman CS. Successful *in utero* therapy of fetal heart block. *Am J Obstet Gynecol* 1995;173:1384

11. Petri M, Golbus M, Anderson R, *et al.* Antinuclear antibody, lupus anticoagulant, and anticardio-lipin antibody in women with idiopathic habitual abortion: a controlled prospective study of 44 women. *Arthr Rheum* 1987;30:601–6

12. Barbui T, Cortelazzo S, Galli M, *et al.* Antiphospholipid antibodies in early repeated abortions: a case-controlled study. *Fertil Steril* 1988;50:589–92

13. Parrazzini F, Acaia B, Faden D, *et al.* Antiphospholipid antibodies and recurrent abortion. *Obstet Gynecol* 1991;77:854–8

14. Parke AL, Wilson D, Maier D. The prevalence of antiphospholipid antibodies in women with recurrent spontaneous abortion, women with successful pregnancies, and women who have never been pregnant. *Arthr Rheum* 1991;34:1231–5

15. Out HJ, Bruinse HW, Christiaens GCML, *et al.* Prevalence of antiphospholipid antibodies in patients with fetal loss. *Ann Rheum Dis* 1991;50:553–7

16. Branch DW, Silver RM, Blackwell JL, Reading JC, Scott JR. Outcome of treated pregnancies in women with antiphospholipid syndrome: an update of the Utah experience. *Obstet Gynecol* 1992;80:61

17. Lima F, Khamashta MA, Buchanan NMM, Kerslake S, Hunt BJ, Hughes GRV. A prospective study of sixty pregnancies in patients with the antiphospholipid syndrome. *Clin Exp Rheumatol* 1996;14:131–6

18. Cowchock FS, Reece EA, Balaban D, Branch DW, Plouffe L. Repeated fetal losses associated with antiphospholipid antibodies: a collaborative randomized trial comparing prednisone with low-dose heparin treatment. *Am J Obstet Gynecol* 1992;166:1318–23

19. Rosove MH, Tabsh K, Wasserstrum N, *et al.* Heparin therapy for pregnant women with lupus anti-coagulant or anticardiolipin antibodies. *Obstet Gynecol* 1990;75:630–4

20. Kutteh WH. Antiphospholipid antibody-associated recurrent pregnancy loss: treatment with hepa-rin and low-dose aspirin is superior to low-dose aspirin alone. *Am J Obstet Gynecol* 1996;174:1584–9

21. Rai R, Cohen H, Dave M, Regan L. Randomised controlled trial of aspirin and aspirin plus heparin in pregnant women with recurrent miscarriage associated with phospholipid antibodies (or antiphospholipid antibodies). *Br Med J* 1997;314:253–7

22. Kerslake S, Morton KE, Versi E, Buchanan NM, Khamashta M, Baguley E, Braude P, Hughes GR. Early Doppler studies in lupus pregnancy. *Am J Reprod Immunol* 1992;28:172–5

23. Farine D, Granovsky-Grisaru S, Ryan G, Seaward PG, Teoh TG, Laskin C, Ritchie JW. Umbilical artery blood flow velocity in pregnancies complicated by systemic lupus erythematosus. *J Clin Ultrasound* 1998;26:379–82

24. Weiner Z, Lorber M, Blumenfeld Z. Umbilical and uterine artery flow velocity waveforms in pregnant women with systemic lupus erythematosus treated with aspirin and glucocorticosteroids. *Am J Reprod Immunol* 1992;28:168–71

25. Guzman E, Schulman H, Bracero L, Rochelson B, Farmakides G, Coury A. Uterine-umbilical artery Doppler velocimetry in pregnant women with systemic lupus erythematosus. *J Ultrasound Med* 1992;11:275–81

26. Caruso A, De Carolis S, Ferrazzani S, Valesini G, Caforio L, Mancuso S. Pregnancy outcome in relation to uterine artery flow velocity waveforms and clinical characteristics in women with antiphospholipid syndrome. *Obstet Gynecol* 1993;82:970–7

27. Trudinger BJ, Stewart GJ, Cook CM, Connelly A, Exner T. Monitoring lupus anticoagulant-positive pregnancies with umbilical artery flow velocity waveforms. *Obstet Gynecol* 1988;72:215–18

28. Carroll BA. Obstetric duplex sonography in patients with lupus anticoagulant syndrome. *J Ultrasound Med* 1990;9:17–21

10

Doppler studies in post-term pregnancies

POST-TERM PREGNANCY

The prevalence of post-term pregnancy (those exceeding 294 days or 42 weeks of gestation) is about 10% when dating is based on the first day of the last menstrual period, but this is only about 5% when dating is by an early ultrasound scan. In about 30% of post-term pregnancies, the fetuses develop a postmaturity syndrome, characterized by growth restriction, dehydration, severe desquamation of the epidermis, bile-stained nails and amnion, advanced hardness of the skull, absence of the vernix caseosa and lanugo hair.

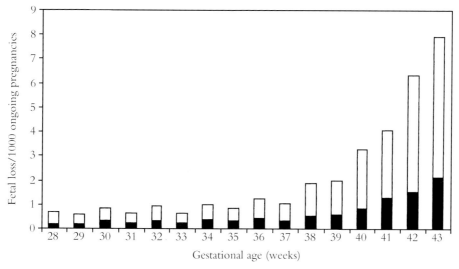

Figure 1   Intrauterine death (black), neonatal death and post-neonatal death (white) per 1000 ongoing pregnancies at each gestation. Adapted by permission from Hilder et al.[1]

Post-term pregnancy is associated with increased risk of both intrauterine and postnatal death. Hilder *et al.* examined 171 527 births in the North East Thames Region in London and reported that the rate of stillbirth increased six-fold from 0.35 per 1000 ongoing pregnancies at 37 weeks of gestation to 2.12 per 1000 pregnancies at 43 weeks (Figure 1). When neonatal and post-neonatal mortality rates are included, the overall risk of death increased from 0.7 per 1000 ongoing pregnancies at 37 weeks to 5.8 per 1000 pregnancies at 43 weeks[1].

There are no morphological features that could indicate an aging process of the term or post-term placenta, either by light or by electron microscopy; furthermore, placental DNA increases linearly with gestation beyond the 40th week of pregnancy[2]. In contrast, the amniotic fluid volume decreases from about 37 weeks, and, during the post-dates period, it is estimated that there is a decrease in amniotic fluid volume of about 33% per week[3,4]. This decrease in amniotic fluid volume, combined with the increased incidence of meconium staining of the amniotic fluid in post-term pregnancies, results in an increased risk of meconium aspiration syndrome. The risk of perinatal death is mainly in the small, postmature, growth-restricted fetus, and the main aim of antenatal monitoring is to identify the onset of uteroplacental insufficiency and the development of fetal hypoxia.

DOPPLER STUDIES

Post-term pregnancies are associated with the development of oligohydramnios and non-reactive fetal heart rate patterns. One possible explanation for the oligohydramnios is decreased fetal renal perfusion due to impaired fetal cardiac function. The alternative hypothesis for the reduction in renal perfusion and urinary output is redistribution in the fetal circulation, as in intrauterine growth restriction. Supportive evidence for impaired fetal renal perfusion as a cause of oligohydramnios in post-term pregnancies was provided by the study of Veille *et al.* who examined 50 pregnancies at or after 40 weeks of gestation. In the 17 with oligohydramnios (amniotic fluid index of less than 5 cm) impedance to flow in the fetal renal artery was significantly higher than in the 33 pregnancies with normal amniotic fluid[5].

Several studies have examined the potential value of Doppler assessment in the prediction of adverse outcome (usually defined as fetal distress in labor) in post-term pregnancies and provided conflicting results (Table 1). All four studies examining uterine arteries reported no significant changes in pregnancies with adverse outcome. Impedance to flow in the umbilical arteries of pregnancies with adverse outcomes was normal in five studies, increased in three studies and decreased in one study. Impedance

Table 1 Studies examining the relation of impedance to flow in the uterine and/or umbilical arteries and fetal cerebral arteries in the prediction of adverse outcome in post-term pregnancies

Author	n	Impedance to flow	Adverse outcome
Rightmire & Campbell, 1987[16]	35	umbilical artery	increased
Brar et al., 1989[19]	45	internal cerebral artery	decreased
Fischer et al., 1991[14]	75	umbilical artery	increased
Anteby et al., 1994[17]	78	umbilical artery	increased
Olofsson et al., 1997[12]	44	umbilical artery	decreased
Anteby et al., 1994[17]	78	middle cerebral artery	decreased
Devine et al., 1994[18]	49	middle cerebral : umbilical artery	decreased
Rightmire & Campbell, 1987[16]	35	uterine artery	normal
Farmakides et al., 1988[20]	149	umbilical and uterine arteries	normal
Brar et al., 1989[19]	45	umbilical and uterine arteries	normal
Stokes et al., 1991[21]	70	umbilical and uterine arteries	normal
Bar-Hava et al., 1995[23]	57	umbilical and middle cerebral arteries	normal
Zimmermann et al., 1995[22]	153	umbilical, uterine and middle cerebral arteries	normal

in the fetal cerebral circulation was reported as being decreased in three studies and normal in two studies.

Impaired fetal cardiac function

There is evidence that the oligohydramnios and abnormal fetal heart rate pattern in post-term fetuses are caused by impaired fetal cardiac function. Thus, Weiner et al. examined 120 post-term pregnancies and reported that the pregnancies with oligo-hydramnios had a significantly lower peak velocity and velocity–time integral in the fetal aortic outflow tract and mitral valve. Post-term fetuses with reduced fetal heart rate variation had a significantly lower peak velocity and velocity–time integral in the aortic and pulmonic outflow tracts and mitral valve[6]. In a further study, Weiner et al. exam-ined 45 pregnancies at 41–43 weeks of gestation. In eight fetuses that subsequently developed an abnormal fetal heart rate pattern in labor, there was a decrease in peak velocity and velocity–time integral in the fetal aortic and pulmonic outflow tracts[7]. It was suggested that, in prolonged pregnancies, cardiac function deteriorates in fetuses that subsequently develop an abnormal fetal heart rate pattern. Similarly, Horenstein et al. examined post-term pregnancies and reported an inverse relationship between fetal ventricular function and amniotic fluid volume[8].

Placental insufficiency and redistribution in the fetal circulation

Battaglia *et al.* compared 16 pregnancies at 40 weeks with 16 pregnancies at more than 41 weeks. In the post-term pregnancies, the time-averaged maximum velocity of the fetal descending thoracic aorta and the ratio of the impedance in the middle cerebral artery to that in the umbilical artery were decreased[9]. Furthermore, post-term pregnancies were associated with an increased incidence of oligohydramnios, increased plasma viscosity and coagulation parameters (decreased fibrinogen, antithrombin III and platelet number). It was concluded that post-term pregnancy may mimic a mild 'fetal growth restriction' [9].

Hitschold *et al.* examined 253 post-term pregnancies for the relation between impedance to flow in the umbilical artery and histological findings in the placenta[10]. Disseminated retarded maturation of the villi was associated with high impedance in the umbilical artery and, in this group, there was a high rate of Cesarean section for fetal distress, low birth weight and high neonatal morbidity. Disseminated retarded maturation of the placenta was found in 66% of the cases with pathological umbilical artery flow velocity waveforms, whereas it occurred only in 6% of the cases with normal flow[10].

Olofsson *et al.* examined 34 pregnancies that delivered after 43 weeks of gestation and reported that, at this gestation, compared to 40 weeks, the mean flow velocity and volume flow in the fetal aorta were lower, the flow velocity in the umbilical vein was higher, impedance to flow in the umbilical artery was lower and impedance to flow in the uterine artery was not different[11]. It was suggested that these findings are compatible with physiological circulatory alterations enhancing continued fetal growth until the late post-term period. There were no signs of any general circulatory deterioration. In a subsequent study, these authors examined 44 pregnancies at 42–43 weeks of gestation. In cases that developed fetal distress in labor, the umbilical artery pulsatility index (PI) was significantly decreased and the fetal aortic volume flow significantly increased; uterine flow was not significantly different. It was suggested that, in post-term pregnancies, subclinical fetal hypoxia may trigger vasodilation of placental vessels (with consequent decrease in umbilical artery PI) and indicates an increase of cardiac output with consequent increased aortic volume flow[12].

Another similarity between the growth-restricted and the post-term fetus was highlighted by the study of Arduini *et al.* who examined the changes in fetal blood flow velocity waveforms during maternal hyperoxygenation[13]. They administered 60% humidified oxygen in 45 post-term pregnancies. During oxygen treatment, nine fetuses exhibited a temporary 20% increase in the impedance to flow in the internal carotid artery and, in this group, there was a higher incidence of emergency Cesarean delivery due to fetal distress and more neonatal complications than in the other 36 fetuses that did not respond to maternal hyperoxygenation. It was concluded that an increase of at least 20% in the PI of the fetal internal carotid artery during maternal hyperoxygenation may be a useful marker of adverse outcome in post-term fetuses.

Some studies reported that the pregnancies which subsequently developed fetal distress in labor were associated with antepartum evidence of increased impedance in the umbilical artery, decreased impedance in the fetal middle cerebral artery, and decreased blood flow velocity in the fetal aorta. Fischer *et al.* examined 75 pregnancies at more than 41 weeks of gestation and reported that impedance to flow in the umbilical artery was significantly higher in those with subsequent abnormal perinatal outcomes than in those with normal outcomes[14]. Similarly, Hitschold *et al.* examined 130 pregnancies at 40–42 weeks of gestation and reported that, in the group with increased impedance in the umbilical artery, the rate of Cesarean section for fetal distress was 53%, compared to 3% in those with normal impedance[15]. Rightmire and Campbell examined 35 pregnancies at more than 42 weeks of gestation and reported that impedance to flow in the uterine and umbilical arteries did not change with gestation, but impedance in the umbilical artery was higher in fetuses with a worse clinical outcome[16]. Blood flow velocity in the fetal descending aorta decreased with gestation and velocity was lower in fetuses who passed meconium before delivery. It was suggested that fetal compromise in prolonged pregnancy is more a fetal–placental problem than a uteroplacental problem[16]. Similarly, Anteby *et al.* examined 78 women at more than 41 weeks of gestation, who had normal non-stress test and amniotic fluid volume[17]. Pregnancies that subsequently developed signs of fetal distress during labor had increased impedance in the umbilical artery, decreased impedance in the fetal middle cerebral artery, and decreased time averaged velocity in the fetal aorta. It was concluded that, in uncomplicated post-term pregnancies, those with abnormal Doppler results are prone to need intervention following fetal distress in labor[17].

Further evidence for centralization of the fetal circulation was provided by the study of Devine *et al.*, who examined 49 pregnancies at more than 41 weeks of gestation and reported that decreased fetal middle cerebral artery to umbilical artery impedance to flow ratio is an accurate method of predicting post-date-related adverse outcome (the occurrence of meconium aspiration syndrome, Cesarean delivery for fetal distress, or fetal acidosis)[18]. A middle cerebral artery to umbilical artery ratio of less than 1.05 predicted an adverse outcome, with a sensitivity of 80%, specificity of 95% and positive predictive value of 80%. In contrast, the sensitivities of oligohydramnios (amniotic fluid index of less than 5 cm), non-reactive fetal heart rate pattern, and a biophysical profile score equal to or less than 6, had sensitivities equal to or less than 40%[18]. Similarly,

Brar *et al.* examined 45 pregnancies at more than 41 weeks of gestation and reported that the incidence of fetal distress in labor was higher in patients with antepartum oligohydramnios (amniotic fluid index less than 5 cm) or non-reactive fetal heart rate pattern. In this group, compared to those with normal amniotic fluid and reactive fetal heart rate pattern, there was no significant difference in impedance to flow in the umbilical and uterine arteries, but impedance in the fetal internal cerebral artery was significantly lower[19].

Normal placental and fetal Doppler

Some studies suggested that the pathophysiology of placental insufficiency in post-term pregnancies differs from that observed in cases of fetal growth restriction at earlier gestational ages, because, in post-term pregnancies, both placental and fetal Doppler indices are normal. Thus, Farmakides *et al.* examined 149 pregnancies at more than 41 weeks of gestation and reported that impedance to flow in the uterine and umbilical arteries was not altered, even in the presence of other signs suggestive of fetal compromise[20]. Similarly, Stokes *et al.* examined 70 pregnancies at more than 41 weeks of gestation and reported that impedance to flow in the umbilical and uteroplacental arteries was not significantly different in pregnancies associated with fetal compromise and abnormal neonatal outcome from those with normal outcome[21].

Zimmermann *et al.* examined 153 pregnancies at 41–43 weeks of gestation and reported that impedance to flow in the umbilical artery, uteroplacental arteries and fetal middle cerebral artery did not change significantly within this gestational range[22]. The majority of Doppler measurements in pregnancies with subsequent asphyxia or otherwise complicated fetal outcome were within the 95% prediction interval for patients with normal fetal outcome. This study also reported that, in the prediction of asphyxia, the sensitivity for oligohydramnios and antepartum cardiotocography was less than 20%.

Bar-Hava *et al.* examined 57 pregnancies at more than 41 weeks of gestation[23]. They measured impedance to flow in the umbilical arteries and the fetal middle cerebral and renal arteries. In 15 pregnancies, there was oligohydramnios and, although in this group the mean birth weight was significantly lower than in the 42 pregnancies with normal amniotic fluid, there were no significant differences between the groups in the Doppler indices. It was concluded that, in post-term pregnancies, oligohydramnios is not associated with a major redistribution in the fetal circulation.

CONCLUSIONS

- Post-term pregnancy is associated with increased risk of both intrauterine and postnatal death.

- In post-term pregnancies, impedance to flow in the uterine arteries is normal.

- In post-term pregnancies with adverse outcomes, impedance to flow in the umbilical arteries may be increased or normal.

- In post-term pregnancies with adverse outcome, impedance to flow in the fetal middle cerebral arteries may be decreased.

- In post-term pregnancies with adverse outcome, blood flow velocity in the fetal descending aorta may be decreased.

- In post-term pregnancies with oligohydramnios, impedance to flow in the fetal renal arteries may be increased.

- In post-term pregnancies with adverse outcome, there is decreased blood flow velocity in fetal aortic and pulmonic outflow tracts and across the mitral valve.

REFERENCES

1. Hilder L, Costeloe K, Thilaganathan B. Prolonged pregnancy: evaluating gestation-specific risks of fetal and infant mortality. *Br J Obstet Gynaecol* 1998;105:169–73

2. Fox H. Placental pathology. In *Progress in Obstetrics and Gynaecology*. Edinburgh: Churchill Livingstone, 1983;3

3. Phelan JP, Platt LD, Yeh SY, Broussard P, Paul RH. The role of ultrasound assessment of amniotic fluid volume in the management of the postdate pregnancy. *Am J Obstet Gynecol* 1985;151:304–8

4. Beischer NA, Brown JB, Townsend L. Studies in prolonged pregnancy. 3. Amniocentesis in prolonged pregnancy. *Am J Obstet Gynecol* 1969;103:496–503

5. Veille JC, Penry M, Mueller-Heubach E. Fetal renal pulsed Doppler waveform in prolonged pregnancies. *Am J Obstet Gynecol* 1993;169:882–4

6. Weiner Z, Farmakides G, Schulman H, Casale A, Itskovitz-Eldor J. Central and peripheral haemodynamic changes in post-term fetuses: correlation with oligohydramnios and abnormal fetal heart rate pattern. *Br J Obstet Gynaecol* 1996;103:541–6

7. Weiner Z, Farmakides G, Barnhard Y, Bar-Hava I, Divon MY. Doppler study of the fetal cardiac function in prolonged pregnancies. *Obstet Gynecol* 1996;88:200–2

8. Horenstein J, Brar H, DeVore G. Cardiovascular evaluation of the post-term fetus. Presented at the *34 Annual Meeting of the Society of Gynaecologic Investigation*, Atlanta, GA, 1987

9. Battaglia C, Artini PG, Ballestri M, Bonucchi D, Galli PA, Bencini S, Genazzani AP. Hemodynamic, hematological and hemorrheological evaluation of post-term pregnancy. *Acta Obstet Gynecol Scand* 1995;74:336–40

10. Hitschold T, Weiss E, Berle P, Muntefering H. Histologic placenta findings in prolonged pregnancy: correlation of placental retarded maturation, fetal outcome and Doppler sonographic findings in the umbilical artery. *Z Geburtshilfe Perinatol* 1989;193:42–6

11. Olofsson P, Saldeen P, Marsal K. Fetal and uteroplacental circulatory changes in pregnancies proceeding beyond 43 weeks. *Early Hum Dev* 1996;46:1–13

12. Olofsson P, Saldeen P, Marsal K. Association between a low umbilical artery pulsatility index and fetal distress in labor in very prolonged pregnancies. *Eur J Obstet Gynecol Reprod Biol* 1997;73:23–9

13. Arduini D, Rizzo G, Romanini C, Mancuso S. Doppler assessment of fetal blood flow velocity waveforms during acute maternal oxygen administration as predictor of fetal outcome in post-term pregnancy. *Am J Perinatol* 1990;7:258–62

14. Fischer RL, Kuhlman KA, Depp R, Wapner RJ. Doppler evaluation of umbilical and uterine-arcuate arteries in the postdates pregnancy. *Obstet Gynecol* 1991;78:363–8

15. Hitschold T, Weiss E, Berle P. Doppler sonography of the umbilical artery, mode of delivery and perinatal morbidity in prolonged pregnancy. *Z Geburtshilfe Perinatol* 1988;192:197–202

16. Rightmire DA, Campbell S. Fetal and maternal Doppler blood flow parameters in postterm pregnancies. *Obstet Gynecol* 1987;69:891–4

17. Anteby EY, Tadmor O, Revel A, Yagel S. Post-term pregnancies with normal cardiotocographs and amniotic fluid columns: the role of Doppler evaluation in predicting perinatal outcome. *Eur J Obstet Gynecol Reprod Biol* 1994;54:93–8

18. Devine PA, Bracero LA, Lysikiewicz A, Evans R, Womack S, Byrne DW. Middle cerebral to umbilical artery Doppler ratio in post-date pregnancies. *Obstet Gynecol* 1994;84:856–60

19. Brar HS, Horenstein J, Medearis AL, Platt LD, Phelan JP, Paul RH. Cerebral, umbilical, and uterine resistance using Doppler velocimetry in postterm pregnancy. *J Ultrasound Med* 1989;8:187–91

20. Farmakides G, Schulman H, Ducey J, Guzman E, Saladana L, Penny B, Winter D. Uterine and umbilical artery Doppler velocimetry in postterm pregnancy. *J Reprod Med* 1988;33:259–61

21. Stokes HJ, Roberts RV, Newnham JP. Doppler flow velocity waveform analysis in postdate pregnancies. *Aust N Z J Obstet Gynaecol* 1991;31:27–30

22. Zimmermann P, Alback T, Koskinen J, Vaalamo P, Tuimala R, Ranta T. Doppler flow velocimetry of the umbilical artery, uteroplacental arteries and fetal middle cerebral artery in prolonged pregnancy. *Ultrasound Obstet Gynecol* 1995;5:189–97

23. Bar-Hava I, Divon MY, Sardo M, Barnhard Y Is oligohydramnios in postterm pregnancy associated with redistribution of fetal blood flow? *Am J Obstet Gynecol* 1995;173:519–22

11

Doppler studies in twin pregnancy

CHORIONICITY IN TWINS

Twins account for about 1% of all pregnancies with two-thirds being dizygotic and one-third monozygotic. All dizygotic pregnancies are dichorionic. In monozygotic pregnancies, splitting of the single embryonic mass into two within 3 days of fertilization, which occurs in one-third of cases, results in dichorionic twins. When embryonic splitting occurs after the 3rd day following fertilization, there are vascular communications within the two placental circulations (monochorionic). Embryonic splitting after the 9th day following fertilization results in monoamniotic monochorionic twins, and splitting after the 12th day results in conjoined twins.

Determination of chorionicity can be performed reliably by ultrasound examination at 11–14 weeks of gestation (Figure 1); in dichorionic twins, there is an extension of placental tissue into the base of the intertwin membrane (lambda sign)[1,2].

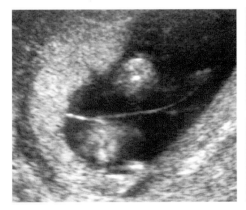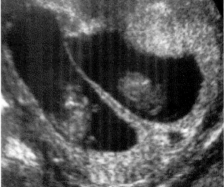

Figure 1 Ultrasound appearance of monochorionic (left) and dichorionic (right) twin pregnancies at 12 weeks of gestation. In both types, there appears to be a single placental mass but, in the dichorionic type, there is an extension of placental tissue into the base of the intertwin membrane, forming the lambda sign

PREGNANCY COMPLICATIONS

In dichorionic twins, the rate of at least one fetal loss between 10 and 24 weeks is about 2.5%, whereas, in monochorionic twins, the rate of fetal loss is about 12%[3]. This increased loss in monochorionic pregnancies is likely to be the consequence of severe early-onset twin-to-twin transfusion syndrome.

The perinatal mortality rate in twins is around six times higher than in singletons, and is about three to four times higher in monochorionic compared to dichorionic twins, regardless of zygosity[4,5]. This increased mortality is mainly due to prematurity-related complications. In a singleton pregnancy, the chance of delivery between 24 and 32 weeks is 1–2%. In monochorionic twins, the incidence is about 9% and in dichorionic twins it is about 5%[3]. In monochorionic twins, an additional complication to prematurity is twin-to-twin transfusion syndrome.

In twin pregnancies, the risk of delivering growth-restricted babies is about ten times higher than in singleton pregnancies[6]. In a study of 467 twin pregnancies, the chance of growth restriction (birth weight below the 5th centile for gestation in single-tons) of at least one of the fetuses was 34% for monochorionic and 23% for dichorionic twins[3]. Furthermore, the chance of growth restriction of both twins was about four times as high in monochorionic (7.5%) compared to dichorionic (1.7%) pregnancies[3]. In monochorionic twins, a disparity in size between the fetuses may be a consequence of the degree of imbalance in fetal nutrition as a result of chronic twin-to-twin trans-fusion syndrome. In dichorionic twins, disparity in size may also be due to differences in fetal nutrition, but in this case such differences may be a consequence of discordancy in the effectiveness of trophoblastic invasion of the maternal spiral arteries and therefore placental function.

Twin-to-twin transfusion syndrome

In monochorionic twin pregnancies, there are placental vascular anastamoses which allow communication of the two fetoplacental circulations[7]. In about 25% of pregnan-cies, imbalance in the net flow of blood across the placental vascular arteriovenous communications from one fetus, the donor, to the other, the recipient, results in twin-to-twin transfusion syndrome; in about half of these cases, there is severe twin-to-twin transfusion syndrome presenting as acute polyhydramnios in the second trimester. The pathognomonic features of severe twin-to-twin transfusion syndrome by ultrasonographic examination are the presence of a large bladder in the polyuric recipient fetus in the polyhydramniotic sac and 'absent' bladder in the anuric donor, that is found to be 'stuck' and immobile at the edge of the placenta or the uterine wall, where it is held fixed by the collapsed membranes of the anhydramniotic sac

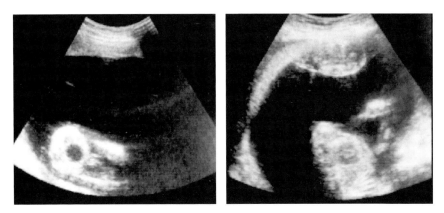

Figure 2 Severe twin-to-twin transfusion syndrome at 20 weeks of gestation. In the polyuric recipient, there is a large bladder and polyhydramnios (left) and the anuric donor is held fixed to the placenta by the collapsed membranes of the anhydramniotic sac (right)

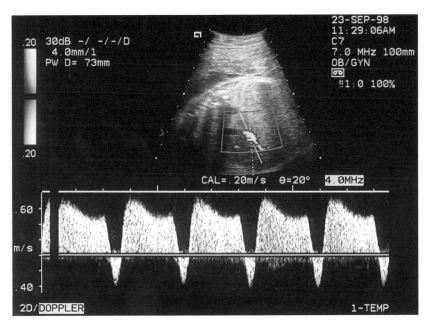

Figure 3 Abnormal waveform of the ductus venosus with reversal of flow during atrial contraction in the recipient fetus of a pregnancy with twin-to-twin transfusion syndrome

(Figure 2)[8]. Other sonographic findings that may prove to be of prognostic significance include the presence of a hypertrophic, dilated and dyskinetic heart, with absence or reversal of flow in the ductus venosus during atrial contraction (Figure 3)[9]. In the donor, the heart may be dilated, the bowel is hyperechogenic, and there is absent end-diastolic flow in the umbilical artery; these features are commonly seen in hypoxemic fetuses in pregnancies with severe uteroplacental insufficiency. In severe twin-to-twin transfusion syndrome, survival with expectant management is less than 10%[8].

The precise underlying mechanisms by which a select population of those monochorionic pregnancies with vascular communications go on to develop twin-to-twin transfusion syndrome is not fully understood. However, it has been hypothesized that primary maldevelopment of the placenta of the donor twin may cause increased peripheral resistance in the placental circulation, which promotes shunting of blood to the recipient; the donor therefore suffers from both hypovolemia due to blood loss and hypoxia due to placental insufficiency[8]. The recipient fetus compensates for its expanded blood volume with polyuria[10], but, since protein and cellular components remain in its circulation, the consequent increase in colloid oncotic pressure draws water from the maternal compartment across the placenta. A vicious cycle of hypervolemia, polyuria, hyperosmolality is established, leading to high-output heart failure and polyhydramnios.

Monoamniotic twins

Splitting of the embryonic mass after day 9 of fertilization results in monoamniotic twins. In these cases, there is a single amniotic cavity with a single placenta and the two umbilical cords insert close to each other. In monoamniotic twins, found in about 1% of all twins or about 5% of monochorionic twins, the fetal loss rate is about 50–75%, due to fetal malformations, preterm delivery and complications arising from the close proximity of the two umbilical cords. Cord entanglement is generally thought to be the underlying mechanism for the majority of fetal losses. However, cord entanglement is found in most cases of monoamniotic twins and this is usually present from the first trimester of pregnancy[11–13]. Therefore, a more likely cause of fetal death in monoamniotic twins, which occurs suddenly and unpredictably, is acute twin-to-twin transfusion syndrome, rather than cord entanglement per se. The close insertion of the umbilical cords into the placenta is associated with large-caliber anastomoses between the two fetal circulations[13,14]. Consequently, an imbalance in the two circulations could not be sustained for prolonged periods of time (which is necessary for the development of the classic features of twin-to-twin transfusion syndrome), but would rather have major hemodynamic effects, causing sudden fetal death.

DOPPLER STUDIES IN TWINS

Several Doppler studies in the 1980s and early 1990s have examined flow velocity waveforms in the umbilical arteries in twin pregnancies[15–24]. These reported that increased impedance provided useful prediction of the subsequent development of fetal growth restriction and adverse perinatal outcome. Furthermore, in pregnancies discordant for growth restriction, there were large intertwin disparities in impedance to flow in the umbilical arteries of the co-twins.

These findings are not surprising, since, in the absence of twin-to-twin transfusion syndrome, the underlying pathophysiology for fetal growth restriction due to placental insufficiency in twins is the same as in singleton pregnancies. Giles *et al.* reported that the histopathological changes in the placentas from twin pregnancies complicated by the presence of abnormal umbilical Doppler results (reduction in the count of small arterial vessels in placental tertiary stem villi restricted to the placenta of the affected fetus) are similar to those found in singleton pregnancies[25].

Neilson *et al.* reported that there were no significant differences between monochorionic and dichorionic pregnancies in either the pattern of umbilical artery flow velocity waveform or intertwin discordance in fetal growth[26]. It was concluded that, in the absence of severe twin-to-twin transfusion syndrome, the vascular anastomoses that have been shown to be common in monochorionic placentas do not exert a strong influence on fetal growth or fetoplacental blood flow.

Two randomized trials of Doppler ultrasound, which included twin pregnancies, have been reported[27,28]. Although the number of twins in these studies was small (16 and 26, and 18 and 22 in the Doppler assessment and control groups, respectively), there was a combined odds ratio of 0.14 (95% confidence interval (CI) 0.03–0.77) for the reduction in fetal death.

Rizzo *et al.* reported that impedance to flow in the uterine arteries is lower in twin than in singleton pregnancies[29]. The diagnostic efficacy of impedance in the uterine artery for predicting the development of gestational hypertension and/or pre-eclampsia was disappointingly low, compared to findings in singleton pregnancies (see Chapter 5).

DOPPLER STUDIES IN TWIN-TO-TWIN TRANSFUSION SYNDROME

Placental vessels

Hecher *et al.* examined the role of color Doppler ultrasonography in the identification of the communicating placental vessels in 18 pregnancies with twin-to-twin transfusion syndrome and two with an acardiac twin[30]. Color Doppler studies of the placental vasculature were performed before fetoscopy for laser coagulation of the communicating vessels. In six cases of twin-to-twin transfusion syndrome, the placental attachment of the intertwin membrane could be visualized, and pulsatile arterial blood flow was observed from the donor to the recipient twin that disappeared after laser therapy. In both cases of acardiac twins, one communicating vessel with pulsatile and another vessel with non-pulsatile blood flow in the opposite direction could be identified. It was suggested that color Doppler imaging is unlikely to play a major role in assisting endoscopic laser separation of chorioangiopagus in patients with acute polyhydramnios, but it may prove to be useful in the early identification of pregnancies at risk of developing twin-to-twin transfusion syndrome.

Denbow *et al.* examined 45 monochorionic pregnancies for the presence of arterio–arterial anastomoses by color Doppler energy[31]. Arterio–arterial anastomoses were present in 8% (1 of 12) that developed twin-to-twin transfusion syndrome, compared to 71% (20 of 28) of those that did not have twin-to-twin transfusion syndrome. It was concluded that twin-to-twin transfusion syndrome is associated with an absence of functional arterio–arterial anastomoses.

Umbilical and fetal arterial Doppler

Giles *et al.* examined 11 pregnancies with twin-to-twin transfusion syndrome (diagnosed retrospectively by the presence of monochorionic placentation and umbilical venous blood hemoglobin differences exceeding 5 g/dl at delivery)[32]. There was no significant difference in the impedance to flow in the umbilical artery between donor and recipient fetuses. In contrast, Pretorius *et al.* examined eight cases of twin-to-twin transfusion syndrome and reported significant differences in umbilical arterial impedance to flow between the fetuses in all cases[33]. However, Doppler studies could not differentiate donor from recipient or provide prognostic data regarding outcome. Yamada *et al.* examined 31 twin pregnancies, including six with twin-to-twin transfusion syndrome[34]. In seven cases, the intertwin difference in umbilical arterial pulsatility index was above 0.5, and, in six of these, there was twin-to-twin transfusion syndrome. Ohno *et al.* reported that, in five pregnancies with twin-to-twin transfusion syndrome, there was intertwin discordancy in umbilical arterial pulsatility index (PI) greater than 0.5 and, in all cases, the PI in the recipient was above the normal range[35]. In contrast, in 28 pregnancies without twin-to-twin transfusion syndrome, there were no cases with increased impedance or discordancy greater than 0.5.

Gaziano *et al.* assessed impedance to flow in the umbilical artery and middle cerebral artery in 33 monochorionic diamniotic twin pregnancies and 50 dichorionic pregnancies[36]. Monochorionic twins demonstrated a significantly greater probability of blood flow redistribution (increased impedance in the umbilical artery and decreased impedance in the middle cerebral artery) than dichorionic twins of similar low birth weights. It was suggested that placental vascular connections and the attendant hemodynamic changes in the fetuses of monochorionic twins may account for this difference.

Hecher *et al.* investigated the circulatory profile of the donor and recipient fetuses in pregnancies with twin-to-twin transfusion syndrome manifested by acute poly-hydramnios during the second trimester of pregnancy[37]. Doppler investigations of the umbilical arteries and of the fetal descending thoracic aortas and middle cerebral arteries were performed in both fetuses of 27 pregnancies with twin-to-twin transfusion syndrome at 18–25 weeks of gestation. Significant differences from normal values were increased umbilical artery PI and decreased aortic mean velocity in both donor and recipient fetuses, decreased middle cerebral artery PI in recipients and decreased middle cerebral artery mean velocity in donors. Increased umbilical artery PI in some donor and recipient fetuses may be the consequence of abnormal placental development and polyhydramnios-related compression, respectively. Doppler findings in the fetal circu-lation are compatible with hypovolemia in the donor and hypervolemia with conges-tive heart failure in the recipient.

Cardiac and venous Doppler

Ishimatsu *et al.* examined 40 twin pregnancies, including six with twin-to-twin trans-fusion syndrome, and reported that the syndrome was not associated with any dis-tinctive findings in umbilical artery blood flow velocity waveforms[38]. However, cardiomegaly in five of the recipient fetuses and tricuspid regurgitation and biphasic umbilical vein waveforms in three recipient fetuses constituted characteristic features of twin-to-twin transfusion syndrome.

Rizzo *et al.* compared Doppler results in 15 dichorionic twin pregnancies (in which the smaller twin subsequently developed antepartum fetal heart rate late decelerations) and ten pregnancies with twin-to-twin transfusion syndrome[39]. Doppler recordings were obtained from umbilical artery, descending aorta, and middle cerebral artery, and the PI was measured. Furthermore, peak velocity from cardiac outflow tract and the percentage of reverse flow in the inferior vena cava were calculated. For all these index values, the intertwin differences (delta value) were determined by subtracting the values obtained in the larger twin from those of the smaller twin. In the dichorionic pregnancies, there were significant changes of delta values for all the parameters tested. In particular, delta values of PI from the umbilical artery and descending aorta progres-sively increased, approaching the occurrence of late decelerations, whereas the delta value for the middle cerebral artery reached a nadir 2 weeks before delivery. Similarly, delta values of peak velocity from outflow tracts significantly decreased, whereas those of the percentage reverse flow in the inferior vena cava increased. In the pregnancies with twin-to-twin transfusion syndrome, there were no significant intertwin differences in PI in any of the vessels that were examined, but there was a significant increase in delta of the peak velocity from the outflow tract and a decrease in the percentage of reverse flow in the inferior vena cava. It was concluded that serial Doppler recordings may show hemodynamic changes in the fetal circulation of discordant twins. Different trends occur according to the underlying pathophysiological mechanisms of the growth defect.

Hecher *et al.* investigated the circulatory profile of the donor and recipient fetuses in 20 pregnancies with twin-to-twin transfusion syndrome presenting with acute polyhydramnios at 17–27 weeks of gestation[9]. Doppler investigations of the arterial vessels and ductus venosus, inferior vena cava, right hepatic vein, tricuspid and mitral ventricular inflow were performed in both fetuses. Mean values of most blood flow velocities on the venous side showed a significant decrease in both groups of fetuses, and a significant increase in mean values for indices describing waveform pulsatility was found in all three venous vessels in the group of recipients, whereas, in the donor group, this was only the case in the ductus venosus. Mean values of atrioventricular flow velocities showed a significant decrease in the donor group. The most significant findings on the arterial side were an increased mean umbilical artery PI and a decreased mean value for aortic blood flow velocity in both groups of fetuses. Five recipients and four donors had absence or reversal of blood flow during atrial contraction in the ductus venosus. All these fetuses showed pulsations in the umbilical vein (Figure 4). Tricuspid regurgitation was present in eight recipients (Figure 5). Absence or reversal of end–diastolic velocities in the umbilical artery was found in four donors. The circulation of the recipient showed the characteristics of congestive heart failure due to hypovolemia. The significant decrease of diastolic venous blood flow velocities is compatible with increased end-diastolic ventricular pressure. Alterations in the circulation of the donor are consistent with decreased venous return due to hypovolemia and increased cardiac afterload due to increased placental resistance.

Zosmer *et al.* examined five pregnancies with twin-to-twin transfusion syndrome and reported increased cardiothoracic ratio and tricuspid regurgitation in all recipient twins[40]. High pulmonary artery velocities developed in three. One recipient twin died a week after delivery of endocardial fibroelastosis and infundibular pulmonary stenosis. Two others had balloon dilatation for pulmonary stenosis, one shortly after birth and one at 4 months. A further twin had apical thickening of the right ventricle at 6 months. The remaining recipient twin had normal echocardiographic findings at follow-up.

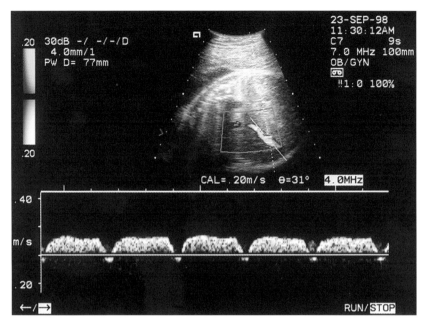

Figure 4 Pulsations in the umbilical vein with reversal of flow at the end of diastole in the recipient fetus of a pregnancy with twin-to-twin transfusion syndrome

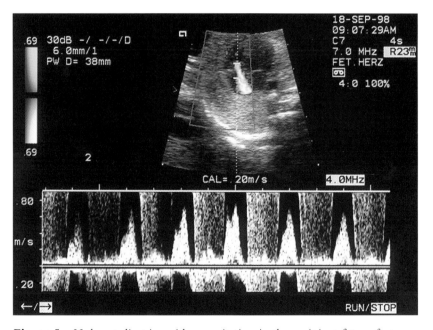

Figure 5 Holosystolic tricuspid regurgitation in the recipient fetus of a pregnancy with twin-to-twin transfusion syndrome

Hecher *et al.* described the sequence of events in the development and subsequent spontaneous resolution of functional tricuspid valve atresia in the donor fetus in a case of twin-to-twin transfusion syndrome[41]. Fetoscopic laser coagulation of the placental anastomoses was performed at 20 weeks of gestation. Subsequently, there was evidence of increased placental vascular resistance in the donor twin and major impairment of right ventricular function, with no forward flow through the tricuspid valve. During the next 4 weeks, however, there was spontaneous and complete recovery of ventricular function and resolution of the functional tricuspid valve atresia. These findings suggest that alterations in fetal hemodynamics may result in structural cardiac abnormality and may be the precursors of some forms of congenital heart disease.

Lachapelle *et al.* examined whether index values of cardiac performance could discriminate between the twin-to-twin transfusion syndrome and placental insufficiency as the etiology of the polyhydramnios–oligohydramnios sequence in monochorionic diamniotic twins, by comparing findings in eight cases with placental insufficiency and five with twin-to-twin transfusion syndrome[42]. Intertwin comparisons were made for the following cardiac parameters: cardiothoracic index, end-diastolic thickness of the ventricular walls and septum, aortic and pulmonary artery Doppler peak velocities, ejection and acceleration times, left ventricular shortening fraction, and combined cardiac output and output indexed to fetal weight. All five recipient twins had thickened ventricular walls. The left ventricular shortening fractions and outputs were significantly increased in the donor twin with twin-to-twin transfusion syndrome and normal in placental insufficiency. It was concluded that, in twin-to-twin transfusion syndrome, the donor twin shows evidence of a hyperdynamic cardiac state. Intertwin comparison of cardiac parameters, especially the left ventricular shortening fraction, can be considered a useful tool in diagnosing the different etiologies of the polyhydramnios–oligohydraminos sequence.

Fesslova *et al.* examined 17 pairs of monochorionic diamniotic twin fetuses with twin-to-twin transfusion syndrome treated by decompressive amniocenteses[43]. Serial Doppler echocardiographic sudies showed no specific cardiac involvement in the donor twins, either *in utero* or after birth. In contrast, all recipient twin fetuses showed variable degrees of biventricular hypertrophy and dilatation with tricuspid regurgitation. These features were evident postnatally but they resolved 1–6 months after birth.

CONCLUSIONS

- In twin pregnancies, impedance to flow in the uterine arteries is lower than in singleton pregnancies.

- In twin pregnancies, impedance to flow in the uterine arteries is not as predictive as in singleton pregnancies of the subsequent development of pre-eclampsia.

- In twin pregnancies, increased impedance to flow in the umbilical arteries provides a useful prediction of the subsequent development of fetal growth restriction and adverse perinatal outcome.

- In twin pregnancies with fetal growth restriction due to placental insufficiency, the growth-restricted fetus demonstrates the same circulatory changes as observed in singleton pregnancies with the same complication. Thus, increased impedance to flow in the umbilical artery is usually associated with arterial redistribution in the fetal circulation, demonstrated by decreased PI in the middle cerebral artery and preferential shift of cardiac output in favor of the left ventricle. Deterioration in the fetal condition is associated with a breakdown of hemodynamic compensatory mechanisms, with a decline in cardiac output and the development of abnormal venous flow with increase in pulsatility of ductus venosus waveforms and loss of forward flow velocity during atrial contraction.

- In pregnancies with twin-to-twin transfusion syndrome, placental vascular anastomoses can be identified by Doppler only in a minority of cases. In monochorionic twins with no twin-to-twin transfusion syndrome, the incidence of vascular anastomoses is much higher than in those with the syndrome.

- In pregnancies with severe twin-to-twin transfusion syndrome, there is increased umbilical artery PI in both the donor and recipient fetuses, which may be the consequence of abnormal placental development and polyhydramnios-related compression, respectively.

- In pregnancies with severe twin-to-twin transfusion syndrome, there is decreased middle cerebral artery PI in recipients and decreased middle cerebral artery mean velocity in donors. Additionally, there is decreased blood flow velocity and increased impedance to flow in the ductus venosus of both the donor and recipient fetuses. In donor fetuses, flow velocities across the atrioventricular valves are decreased. In a high proportion of recipient fetuses, there is tricuspid regurgitation.

- In pregnancies with severe twin-to-twin transfusion syndrome, Doppler findings in the fetal circulation of the donor are consistent with decreased venous return due to hypovolemia and increased cardiac afterload due to increased placental resistance. In the recipient, there is evidence of hypervolemia with congestive heart failure; hypervolemia may cause compensatory cardiac hypertrophy, but eventually the pumping capabilities of the enlarged heart are exceeded and cardiac failure occurs.

REFERENCES

1. Bessis R, Papiernik E. Echographic imagery of amniotic membranes in twin pregnancies. In Gedda L, Parisi P, eds. *Twin Research 3: Twin Biology and Multiple Pregnancy.* New York: Alan R Liss, 1981:183–7

2. Sepulveda W, Sebire NJ, Hughes K, Odibo A, Nicolaides KH. The lambda sign at 10–14 weeks of gestation as a predictor of chorionicity in twin pregnancies. *Ultrasound Obstet Gynecol* 1996;7:421–3

3. Sebire NJ, Snijders RJM, Hughes K, Sepulveda W, Nicolaides KH. The hidden mortality of monochorionic twin pregnancies. *Br J Obstet Gynaecol* 1997;104:1203–7

4. Derom R, Vlietnick R, Derom C, Thiery M, Van Maele G, Van den Berghe H. Perinatal mortality in the East Flanders prospective twin survey. *Eur J Obstet Gynecol* 1991;41:25–6

5. Machin G, Bamforth F, Innes M, Minichul K. Some perinatal characteristics of monozygotic twins who are dichorionic. *Am J Med Genet* 1995;55:71–6

6. Luke B, Keith LG. The contribution of singletons, twins and triplets to low birth weight, infant mortality and handicap in the United States. *J Reprod Med* 1992;37:661–6

7. Benirschke K. Twin placenta in perinatal mortality. *N Y St J Med* 1961;61:1499–508

8. Saunders NJ, Snijders RJM, Nicolaides KH. Therapeutic amniocentesis in twin–twin transfusion syndrome appearing in the second trimester of pregnancy. *Am J Obstet Gynecol* 1992;166:820–4

9. Hecher K, Ville Y, Snijders R, Nicolaides KH. Doppler studies of the fetal circulation in twin–twin transfusion syndrome. *Ultrasound Obstet Gynecol* 1995 5:318–24

10. Rosen D, Rabinowitz R, Beyth Y, Feijgin MD, Nicolaides KH. Fetal urine production in normal twins and in twins with acute polyhydramnios. *Fetal Diagn Ther* 1990;5:57–60

11. Rodis JF, McIlveen PF, Egan JF, Borgida AF, Turner GW, Campbell WA. Monoamniotic twins: improved perinatal survival with accurate prenatal diagnosis and antenatal fetal surveillance. *Am J Obstet Gynecol* 1997;177:1046–9

12. Overton TG, Denbow ML, Duncan KR, Fisk NM. First-trimester cord entanglement in monoamniotic twins. *Ultrasound Obstet Gynecol* 1999;13:140–2

13. Arabin B, Laurini RN, Van Eyck J. Early prenatal diagnosis of cord entanglement in monoamniotic multiple pregnancies. *Ultrasound Obstet Gynecol* 1999;13:181–6

14. Bajoria R. Abundant vascular anastamoses in monoamniotic versus diamniotic monochorionic placentas. *Am J Obstet Gynecol* 1998;179:788–93

15. Giles WB, Trudinger BJ, Cook CM. Fetal umbilical artery flow velocity-time waveforms in twin pregnancies. *Br J Obstet Gynaecol* 1985;92:490–7

16. Farmakides G, Schulman H, Saldana LR, Bracero LA, Fleischer A, Rochelson B. Surveillance of twin pregnancy with umbilical arterial velocimetry. *Am J Obstet Gynecol* 1985;153:789–92

17. Gerson AG, Wallace DM, Bridgens NK, Ashmead GG, Weiner S, Bolognese RJ. Duplex Doppler ultrasound in the evaluation of growth in twin pregnancies. *Obstet Gynecol* 1987;70:419–23

18. Nimrod C, Davies D, Harder J, Dempster C, Dodd G, McDicken N, Nicholson S. Doppler ultrasound prediction of fetal outcome in twin pregnancies. *Am J Obstet Gynecol* 1987;156:402–6

19. Divon MY, Girz BA, Sklar A, Guidetti DA, Langer O. Discordant twins – a prospective study of the diagnostic value of real-time ultrasonography combined with umbilical artery velocimetry. *Am J Obstet Gynecol* 1989;161:757–60

20. Hastie SJ, Danskin F, Neilson JP, Whittle MJ. Prediction of the small for gestational age twin fetus by Doppler umbilical artery waveform analysis. *Obstet Gynecol* 1989;74:730–3

21. Gaziano EP, Knox GE, Bendel RP, Calvin S, Brandt D. Is pulsed Doppler velocimetry useful in the management of multiple-gestation pregnancies? *Am J Obstet Gynecol* 1991;164:1426–33

22. Degani S, Gonen R, Shapiro I, Paltiely Y, Sharf M. Doppler flow velocity waveforms in fetal surveillance of twins: a prospective longitudinal study. *J Ultrasound Med* 1992;11:537–41

23. Kurmanavicius J, Hebisch G, Huch R, Huch A. Umbilical artery blood flow velocity waveforms in twin pregnancies. *J Perinat Med* 1992;20:307–12

24. Jensen OH. Doppler velocimetry in twin pregnancy. *Eur J Obstet Gynecol Reprod Biol* 1992;45:9–12

25. Giles W, Trudinger B, Cook C, Connelly A. Placental microvascular changes in twin pregnancies with abnormal umbilical artery waveforms. *Obstet Gynecol* 1993;81:556–9

26. Neilson JP, Danskin F, Hastie SJ. Monozygotic twin pregnancy: diagnostic and Doppler ultrasound studies. *Br J Obstet Gynaecol* 1989;96:1413–18

27. Omtzigt AWJ. *Clinical value of umbilical Doppler velocimetry; randomized controlled trial*. Doctoral thesis, University of Utrecht, 1990

28. Johnstone FD, Prescott R, Hoskins, Greer IA, McGlew T, Compton M. The effect of introduction of umbilical Doppler recordings to obstetric practice. *Br J Obstet Gynaecol* 1993;100:733–41

29. Rizzo G, Arduini D, Romanini C. Uterine artery Doppler velocity waveforms in twin pregnancies. *Obstet Gynecol* 1993;82:978–83

30. Hecher K, Ville Y, Nicolaides KH. Color Doppler ultrasonography in the identification of communicating vessels in twin–twin transfusion syndrome and acardiac twins. *J Ultrasound Med* 1995;14:37–40

31. Denbow ML, Cox P, Talbert D, Fisk NM. Colour Doppler energy insonation of placental vasculature in monochorionic twins: absent arterio–arterial anastomoses in association with twin-to-twin transfusion syndrome. *Br J Obstet Gynaecol* 1998;105:760–5

32. Giles WB, Trudinger BJ, Cook CM, Connelly AJ. Doppler umbilical artery studies in the twin–twin transfusion syndrome. *Obstet Gynecol* 1990;76:1097–9

33. Pretorius DH, Manchester D, Barkin S, Parker S, Nelson TR. Doppler ultrasound of twin transfusion syndrome. *J Ultrasound Med* 1988;7:117–24

34. Yamada A, Kasugai M, Ohno Y, Ishizuka T, Mizutani S, Tomoda Y. Antenatal diagnosis of twin–twin transfusion syndrome by Doppler ultrasound. *Obstet Gynecol* 1991;78:1058–61

35. Ohno Y, Ando H, Tanamura A, Kurauchi O, Mizutani S, Tomoda Y. The value of Doppler ultrasound in the diagnosis and management of twin-to-twin transfusion syndrome. *Arch Gynecol Obstet* 1994;255:37–42

36. Gaziano E, Gaziano C, Brandt D. Doppler velocimetry determined redistribution of fetal blood flow: correlation with growth restriction in diamniotic monochorionic and dizygotic twins. *Am J Obstet Gynecol* 1998;178:1359–67

37. Hecher K, Ville Y, Nicolaides KH. Fetal arterial Doppler studies in twin–twin transfusion syndrome. *J Ultrasound Med* 1995;14:101–8

38. Ishimatsu J, Yoshimura O, Manabe A, Matsuzaki T, Tanabe R, Hamada T. Ultrasonography and Doppler studies in twin-to-twin transfusion syndrome. *Asia Oceania J Obstet Gynaecol* 1992;18: 325–31

39. Rizzo G, Arduini D, Romanini C. Cardiac and extracardiac flows in discordant twins. *Am J Obstet Gynecol* 1994;170:1321–7

40. Zosmer N, Bajoria R, Weiner E, Rigby M, Vaughan J, Fisk NM. Clinical and echographic features of *in utero* cardiac dysfunction in the recipient twin in twin–twin transfusion syndrome. *Br Heart J* 1994;72:74–9

41. Hecher K, Sullivan ID, Nicolaides KH. Temporary iatrogenic fetal tricuspid valve atresia in a case of twin to twin transfusion syndrome. *Br Heart J* 1994;72:457–60

42. Lachapelle MF, Leduc L, Cote JM, Grignon A, Fouron JC. Potential value of fetal echocardiography in the differential diagnosis of twin pregnancy with presence of polyhydramnios–oligohydramnios syndrome. *Am J Obstet Gynecol* 1997;177:388–94

43. Fesslova V, Villa L, Nava S, Mosca F, Nicolini U. Fetal and neonatal echocardiographic findings in twin–twin transfusion syndrome. *Am J Obstet Gynecol* 1998;179:1056–62

12

Color Doppler sonography in the assessment of the fetal heart

Rabih Chaoui

INTRODUCTION

Pulsed and color Doppler ultrasound improve the diagnostic accuracy of two-dimensional gray-scale imaging in the prenatal detection of abnormalities of the heart and great arteries. The two methods are complementary to each other, with color Doppler being used for general assessment of flow in the region of interest and pulsed Doppler for targeted examination of flow in a vessel or across a valve[1–10].

In pulsed Doppler ultrasound, the examiner positions a sample volume over the region of interest to obtain flow velocity waveforms as a function of time. This makes it possible to quantify blood flow as peak or time-averaged mean velocities, which allow the calculation of ratios (such as the E/A ratio) or blood volume (such as stroke volume or cardiac output) after measurement of vessel diameter. Color Doppler, which is technically easier to perform, allows a rapid assessment of the hemodynamic situation, but gives only descriptive or semi-quantitative information on blood flow. Color Doppler should be an integral part of the routine examination of a fetal heart because this helps to shorten the scanning time, but also provides improved reliability in diagnosing or excluding abnormalities.

EXAMINATION OF THE NORMAL HEART

Examination of the fetal heart using color Doppler is achieved through similar planes as gray-scale imaging. Several planes, including the abdominal view, four-chamber view, five-chamber view, the short-axis and the three-vessel view need to be assessed to achieve spatial information on different cardiac chambers and vessels as well as their

171

connections to each other[1,2,4]. The difference from two-dimensional scanning is that, with color Doppler, the angle of insonation should be as small as possible for optimal visualization of flow.

In the abdominal plane, the position of the aorta, inferior vena cava and the connection of the vein to the right atrium are examined. Pulsed Doppler sampling from the inferior vena cava, the ductus venosus or the hepatic veins can be achieved in longitudinal planes.

The four-chamber view allows the detection of many severe cardiac defects. Using color Doppler in an apical (Figure 1) or basal approach, the diastolic perfusion across the atrioventricular valves can be assessed; there is a characteristic separate perfusion of both inflow tracts during diastole (Figure 1). Using pulsed Doppler, there is a typical biphasic shape of the diastolic flow velocity waveform with an early peak diastolic velocity (E) and a second peak during atrial contraction (A-wave); E is smaller than A, and the E : A ratio increases during pregnancy toward 1, to be inversed after birth. In this plane, regurgitation across the atrioventricular valves, which is more frequent at the tricuspid valve, is easily detected during systole with color Doppler. Flow across the foramen

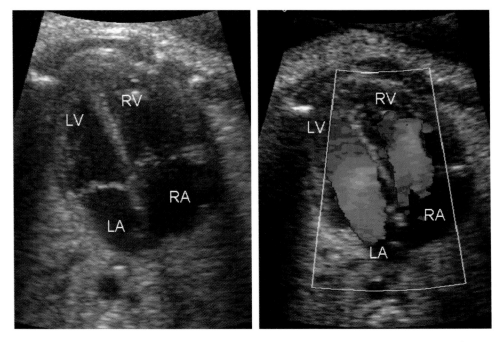

Figure 1 Four-chamber view in real-time (left) and color Doppler. During diastole, flow is visualized entering from both the right and left atria (RA, LA) into the right and left ventricles (RV, LV) and the flows are separated by the interatrial and interventricular septum

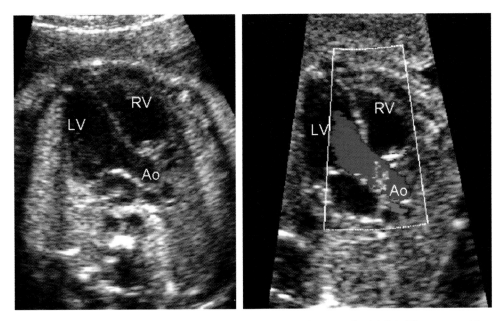

Figure 2 Five-chamber view in real-time (left) using color Doppler (right). The aorta, arising from the left ventricle, is seen and color shows the laminar flow across the aortic valve during systole. Compare with aortic stenosis (Figure 7) and overriding aorta (Figure 12)

ovale is visualized in a lateral approach of the four-chamber view. Color Doppler allows confirmation of the physiological right-to-left shunt and visualization of the pulmonary veins as they enter the left atrium.

The transducer is then tilted to obtain the five-chamber view and then the short-axis view. Using color Doppler, flow during systole is visualized (Figure 2). In these planes, the correct ventriculo–arterial connections (compare Figures 2 and 14), the non-aliased flow (compare Figures 2 and 7) and the continuity of the interventricular septum with the aortic root are examined (compare Figures 2 and 12). With pulsed Doppler, a single peak flow velocity waveform for the aortic and pulmonary valves is demonstrated. The peak systolic velocity increases from 50 to 110 cm/s during the second half of pregnancy and is higher across the aortic than the pulmonary valve. Time to peak velocity in the aorta is longer than in the pulmonary trunk.

The three-vessel view enables assessment of the aortic arch and the ductus arteriosus. In the third trimester, an aliased flow is found within the ductus as a sign of the onset of constriction. When the fetal position is optimal, the aortic arch and ductus arteriosus can be seen in a longitudinal plane, allowing visualization of neck vessels.

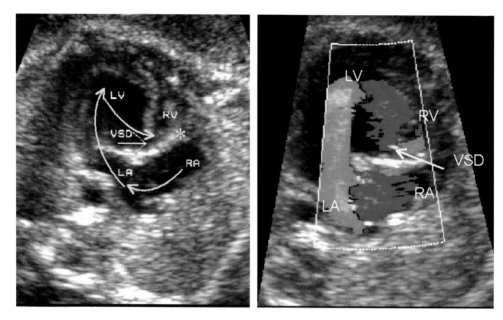

Figure 3 Tricuspid atresia (★) and ventricular septal defect (VSD). Arrows show the direction of flow; due to the atresia of the tricuspid valve, blood entering the right atrium cannot enter directly into the right ventricle and it flows to the left atrium, left ventricle and across the VSD to the hypoplastic right ventricle (right)

EXAMINATION OF THE ABNORMAL HEART

Tricuspid atresia

In this condition, there is absence of the connection between the right atrium and the right ventricle. In the four-chamber view, the right ventricle is hypoplastic or absent and color Doppler demonstrates the absence of flow from the right atrium to the right ventricle (Figure 3). Blood from the right atrium flows across the foramen ovale to the left atrium and from there during diastole to the left ventricle. This unilateral perfusion across the left ventricular inflow tract is typical for this lesion. In the presence of an associated ventricular septal defect, a left-to-right shunt into the small right ventricular cavity is found. The postnatal prognosis depends on the anatomy of the great vessels. The ventriculo–arterial connection can be concordant or discordant, and the pulmonary valve can be patent, stenotic or atretic; color Doppler helps in the reliable differentiation between these conditions.

Tricuspid dysplasia and Ebstein anomaly

In tricuspid dysplasia, the valve leaflets are correctly inserted but they are thickened. By contrast, the valve leaflets in Ebstein anomaly are inserted abnormally so that they are more apical in the right ventricle and their ability to close is reduced. In both conditions there is tricuspid regurgitation which is generally associated with dilatation of the right atrium and, in extreme forms, with gross cardiomegaly (Figure 4)[11,12]. Color Doppler is used to confirm tricuspid regurgitation and spectral Doppler (Figure 5) is used to measure the pressure gradient and duration of the regurgitation. Since both anomalies are associated with an obstruction of the right ventricular outflow tract (pulmonary stenosis or atresia), it is mandatory to analyze the perfusion in the pulmonary trunk. In severe obstruction, retrograde flow within the ductus arteriosus is found (see Figure 6). This, however, does not prove pulmonary atresia because a patent but stenotic pulmonary valve, due to tricuspid regurgitation, can show the same features as an atresia and thus leads to a false-positive result[12].

Pulmonary atresia and intact ventricular septum

This diagnosis includes a group of heart defects with an atretic pulmonary valve and an intact ventricular septum. The size and shape of the right ventricle show a wide range, from hypoplastic to normal sized or even dilated. The latter form is identical to tricuspid dysplasia with pulmonary atresia. In both former types, the right ventricle shows no contractility and the tricuspid valve movements are reduced. Color Doppler in the four-chamber view shows absence or reduced tricuspid flow and, during systole, there may be tricuspid valve regurgitation. In the three-vessel view or the short-axis view,

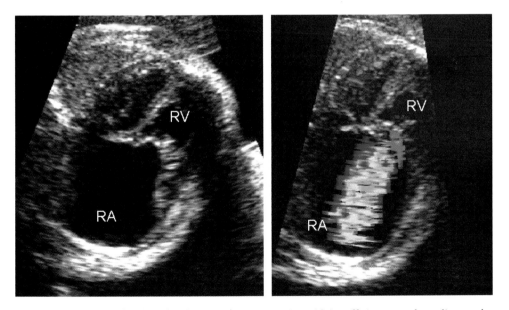

Figure 4 Tricuspid valve dysplasia with severe tricuspid insufficiency and cardiomegaly. Retrograde flow from the right ventricle (RV) to the right atrium (RA) is seen in blue and turbulence is coded by green pixels

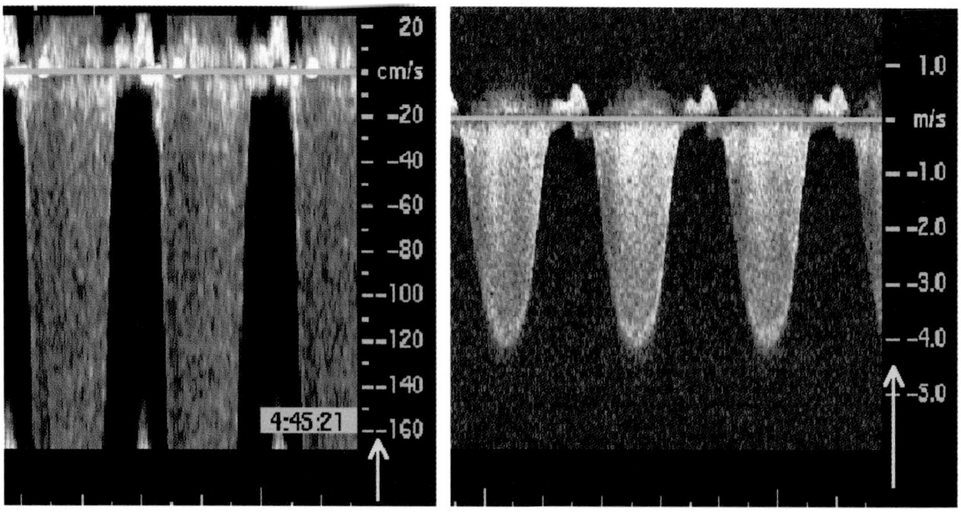

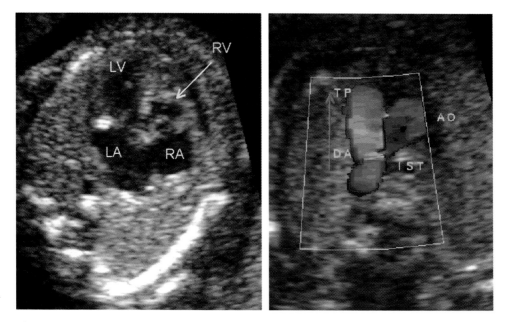

Figure 5 Severe tricuspid regurgitation. Pulsed wave Doppler (left) is not useful due to the aliasing phenomenon and the maximal velocities that can be assessed are 180 cm/s (arrow). The continuous wave transducer allows assessment of very high velocities; in this case 420 cm/s

Figure 6 Hypoplastic right ventricle (arrow) in a fetus with pulmonary atresia and intact ventricular septum. Pulmonary valve atresia can be diagnosed using color Doppler by visualizing the great vessels – aorta (Ao) and pulmonary trunk (TP) – in the upper thorax and demonstrating the retrograde flow from the descending aorta across the ductus arteriosus toward the pulmonary valve

there is absence of antegrade perfusion across the pulmonary valve and retrograde flow through the ductus arteriosus (Figure 6). The pulmonary trunk in these conditions is narrower than the ascending aorta, but is not severely hypoplastic because of retrograde perfusion through the ductus arteriosus. In some hearts with pulmonary atresia, communications between the hypoplastic right ventricle and the coronary arteries may be present and are detectable by color Doppler ultrasound[13] in mid-gestation. Their presence is associated with worse neonatal outcome.

Pulmonary stenosis

In the isolated form of this lesion, there is narrowing of the semilunar valves. In severe cases, a hypokinetic and hypertrophied right ventricle can be found but most cases are not detected prenatally. On two-dimensional imaging, the diagnosis is suspected by the presence of poststenotic dilatation of the pulmonary trunk and reduction of pulmonary valve excursion. With color Doppler, the diagnosis is easy and is based on the demonstration of turbulent flow across the pulmonary valve. In severe cases, a retrograde flow can be found through the ductus arteriosus. Doppler flow velocity waveforms using a continuous wave transducer enable the demonstration of high velocities (more than 2 m/s), which are typical of stenosis. These findings, either in color or in pulsed Doppler, are only typical of the isolated form and are not commonly found in conditions associated with a ventricular septal defect, such as tetralogy of Fallot or double outlet right ventricle. Fetal pulmonary stenosis can be associated in the third trimester with tricuspid insufficiency, leading in some cases to right atrial dilatation[8].

Aortic stenosis

In general, the narrowing is found at the level of the aortic valve and a simple stenosis is rarely detected in the four-chamber view. However, a critical aortic stenosis is associated with a dilated and hypokinetic left ventricle with an echogenic endocardium, as a sign of endocardial fibroelastosis. Simple aortic stenosis can be detected only by using color Doppler (Figure 7). Antegrade turbulent flow (aliasing) is a characteristic finding in the five-chamber view (Figure 7). Pulsed Doppler analysis shows high velocities (more than 2 m/s) and a characteristic aliasing pattern. Continuous wave Doppler is therefore necessary to confirm the diagnosis (Figure 7). In critical aortic stenosis, there is antegrade turbulent flow across the aortic valve, but peak systolic velocities can vary from more than 2 m/s to values within the normal range, as an expression of left ventricular dysfunction[9]. Due to the high pressure in the left ventricle, both a mitral regurgitation and a left-to-right shunt at the level of the foramen ovale are found[8]. In severe left ventricular dysfunction, a retrograde flow is seen within the aortic arch.

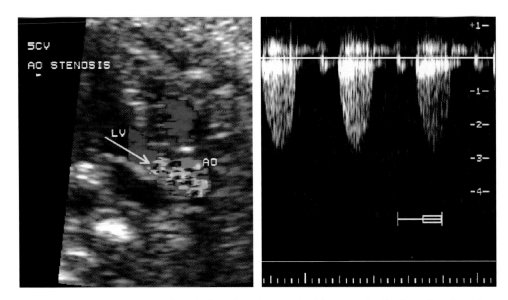

Figure 7 Aortic stenosis with turbulent flow (green pixels), as seen in the five-chamber view (compare with normal findings in Figure 2). Continuous wave Doppler allows a quantification of the stenosis

Hypoplastic left heart syndrome

In this condition, the aortic valve is generally atretic or severely stenotic and the left ventricle diminutive and non-contractile. The mitral valve is either atretic (Figure 8) or stenotic (Figure 9). Color Doppler demonstrates reduced or absent diastolic filling of the left ventricle[8]. In the four-chamber view, there is unilateral perfusion of the right ventricle. Often, there is mild tricuspid regurgitation. Careful examination of the intra-atrial communication shows an abnormal left-to-right shunt. In hypoplastic left heart syndrome, there is retrograde perfusion of the neck vessels and coronary arteries which can also be used for the differential diagnosis[14,15]. Using color Doppler, it is then possible to confirm the diagnosis by demonstrating, in the three-vessel view, the retrograde perfusion in the hypoplastic aortic arch[14,15].

Ventricular septal defect

The defect can be either situated in the inlet, in the muscular part or, most commonly, in the perimembranous part of the ventricular septum. The defect can be suspected by two-dimensional ultrasound examination if it is larger than 3 mm. Color Doppler can help to identify small muscular septal defects (Figure 10). Although right and left ventricular pressures are quite equal prenatally, a bidirectional shunt across the defect is present. The best approach to examine a septal defect with color Doppler is the

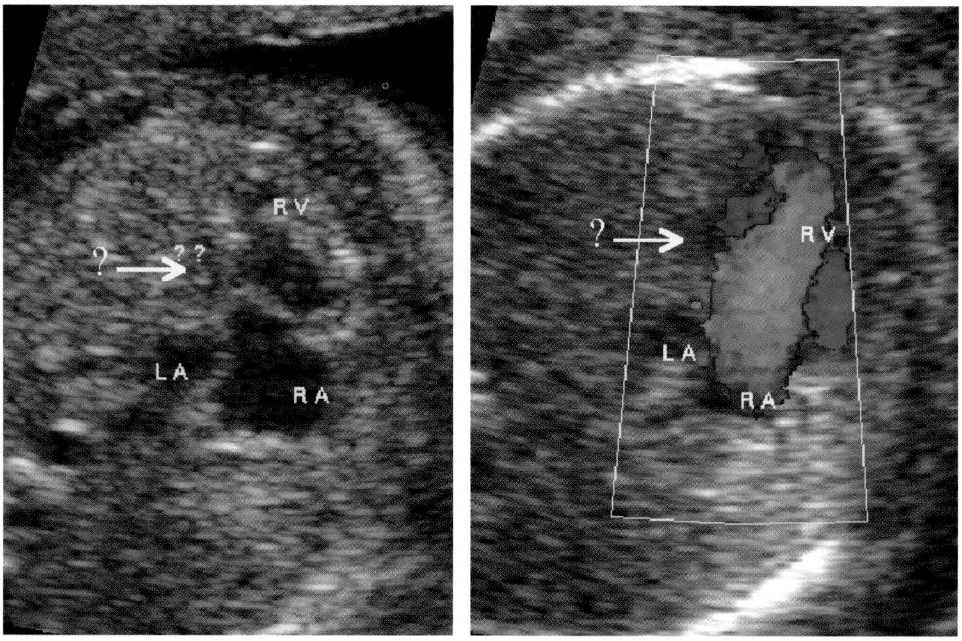

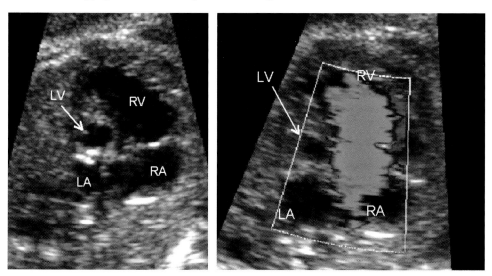

Figure 8 Hypoplastic left heart syndrome. The left ventricle (LV) is absent (?) due to mitral atresia and aortic atresia. Color Doppler shows the one-sided perfusion from the right atrium into the right ventricle (RA, RV). Compare with the normal four-chamber view in Figure 1 and with another hypoplastic left heart syndrome in Figure 9

Figure 9 Hypoplastic left heart syndrome. In comparison with the fetus in Figure 8, this fetus shows a hypoplastic hypokinetic left ventricle. This is due to the combination of aortic atresia and patent but dysplastic mitral valve. Color Doppler shows similar features as in Figure 8, with one-sided perfusion across the right ventricular inflow tract

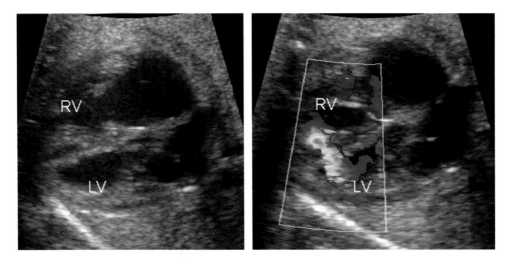

Figure 10 Four-chamber view seen from the right side. With real-time scanning, the anatomy appears to be normal. The use of color Doppler demonstrates the presence of a muscular ventricular septal defect during the phase of a shunt (blue) between the right and left ventricles

perpendicular insonation of the interventricular septum (Figure 10). In cases of an obstruction of an outflow tract, there is an unidirectional shunt to the contralateral side; in a ventricular septal defect with aortic stenosis, there is a left–to–right shunt[8].

Atrioventricular septal defect

In this malformation, there is a combination of defects in the atrial and ventricular septum at the level of the atrioventricular connections. The septal valve leaflets are generally malformed and, in severe cases, they can be absent. In a complete atrioventricular septal defect, color Doppler produces a characteristic H-shape with biventricular diastolic flow across the right and the left inflow tracts and a communication at the level of the atrioventricular valves (Figure 11)[6]. During systole, the dysplastic valves are not able to close properly, leading to tricuspid and mitral regurgitation (Figure 12). If the regurgitation is severe, cardiac failure and non-immune hydrops develop[16].

Tetralogy of Fallot

This cardiac defect is defined by the association of a ventricular septal defect, an overriding aorta, an infundibular pulmonary stenosis and a secondary hypertrophy of the right ventricle. Prenatally, the first three signs are present and they can be diagnosed. Using two-dimensional ultrasound, the ventricular septal defect and overriding aorta

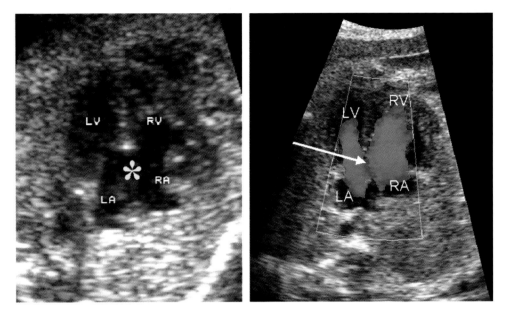

Figure 11 Four-chamber view in a fetus with Down syndrome demonstrating a complete atrioventricular septal defect (AV canal). The defect (★) can be recognized during diastole when the valves are patent but is better assessed using color Doppler, which demonstrates the interatrial and interventricular connection during diastole (H-shape). Compare with the normal findings in Figure 1

can be seen in the five-chamber view. With color Doppler, the Y-shape of systolic blood flow from both ventricles into the overriding aorta can be visualized (Figure 13)[6]. However, an overriding vessel is not exclusive to tetralogy of Fallot, as it can be found in truncus arteriosus communis, in some forms of double outlet right ventricle or in pulmonary atresia with ventricular septal defect. It is, therefore, important to assess the anatomy and hemodynamics of the pulmonary trunk, when an overriding vessel is suspected.

Double outlet right ventricle

This is a group of cardiac defects in which the aorta and pulmonary trunk originate from the right ventricle. The position of these vessels to each other is variable, but they usually have a parallel course. In most cases, the diagnosis is achieved using two-dimensional ultrasound, but this is often facilitated by applying color Doppler (Figure 14). In hearts with double outlet right ventricle, obstructions of the pulmonary or aortic pathway can be present and are easily diagnosed by color Doppler. In patent atrioventricular valves, the left ventricle appears smaller than the right one and flow across the ventricular septal defect is found to be unidirectional from left to right.

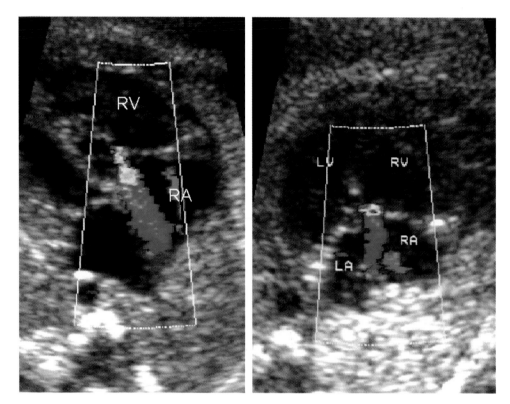

Figure 12 Regurgitation of the tricuspid valve. On the left, trivial regurgitation and, on the right, valve regurgitation in a fetus with an atrioventricular septal defect

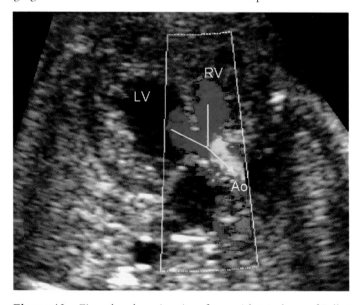

Figure 13 Five-chamber view in a fetus with tetralogy of Fallot (TOF), demonstrating the systolic perfusion from both the right and left ventricle (RV, LV) into the overriding aorta (Y-shape)

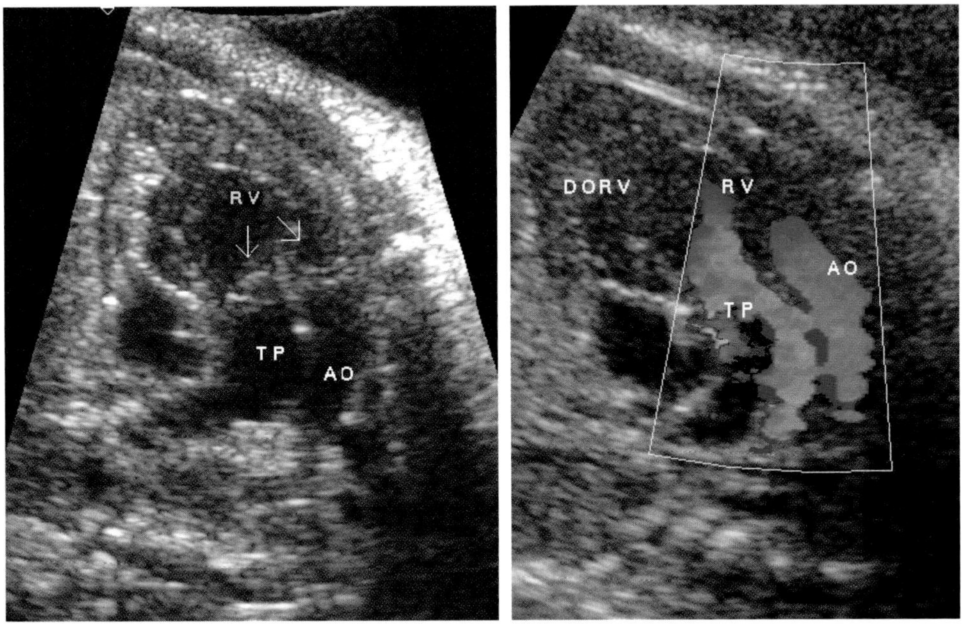

Figure 14 Double outlet right ventricle (DORV) with both the aorta (AO) and pulmonary trunk (TP) arising from the right ventricle. Color Doppler demonstrates blood flow from the right ventricle into both vessels and the flow is not turbulent because there is no stenosis

Complete transposition of the great arteries

In this defect, the aorta arises from the right ventricle and the pulmonary trunk from the left ventricle. The diagnosis is suspected postnatally when the infant becomes cyanotic after closure of the ductus arteriosus and foramen ovale. Prenatally, the four-chamber view appears normal. The malformation is recognized when both arteries are visualized simultaneously and they appear to be parallel to each other (Figure 15); color Doppler is particularly helpful in demonstrating this sign. Color Doppler is also useful in demonstrating pulmonary stenosis and ventricular septal defect, which are occasionally found in transposition of the great arteries.

Other heart defects

Color Doppler is useful in the diagnosis of a wide range of fetal heart defects, including abnormal connections of systemic or pulmonary veins, truncus arteriosus communis, anomalies of the aortic arch, and assessment of intracardiac hemodynamics in cardiomyopathies or in cardiac tumors.

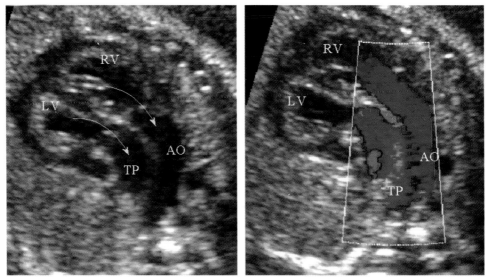

Figure 15 Transposition of the great arteries demonstrating the abnormal connection of the right ventricle (RV) with the aorta (AO) and the left ventricle (LV) with the pulmonary trunk (TP). Both great arteries show a parallel course

DIFFERENTIAL DIAGNOSIS OF TRICUSPID REGURGITATION

Regurgitation of the fetal atrioventricular valves is more common on the right side than on the left. Regurgitation of the tricuspid valve shows a wide range of severity, from harmless regurgitation of short duration[15] to severe insufficiency lasting throughout the whole of systole (holosystolic), leading to huge dilatation of the right atrium (Figure 4). In some conditions, gross dilatation of the right atrium can be the first sign detected on real-time imaging[11] and targeted color Doppler demonstrates severe insufficiency to be the underlying cause. On many occasions, however, tricuspid regurgitation is detected accidently when performing either a routine examination with color Doppler or during a targeted fetal echocardiographic scan in suspected fetal disease. Tricuspid regurgitation of short duration in early systole is observed in 3–5% of all healthy fetuses at mid-gestation[17,18] and this is considered to be physiological. However, the detection of tricuspid regurgitation should stimulate a search for a possible underlying pathology (Table 1).

Table 1   Differential diagnosis of fetal tricuspid regurgitation

Pathogenesis	Etiology
Mild regurgitation	physiological due to immature fetal lungs or myocardium. Found in 3–5% of all pregnancies at 18–24 weeks
Heart defects with dysplasia of the tricuspid valve	Ebstein anomaly tricuspid valve dysplasia
Heart defects with facultative tricuspid regurgitation	atrioventricular valve septal defect hypoplastic left heart syndrome coarctation of the aorta double outlet right ventricle
Heart defects and diseases with right ventricular outflow tract obstruction	pulmonary atresia pulmonary stenosis constriction of the ductus arteriosus (mild to severe tricuspid regurgitation
Volume overload (often with mitral regurgitation)	fetal anemia, due to red cell isoimmunization, parvovirus B19 infection, fetomaternal hemorrhage peripheral arteriovenous fistula, due to a vein of Galen aneurysm, sacrococcygeal teratoma, chorangioma severe tachycardia or bradycardia recipient fetus in twin-to-twin transfusion syndrome heart defect with volume overload or pulmonary regurgitation (tetralogy of Fallot with absent pulmonary valve)
Impairment of myocardial contractility	myocarditis, due to infection, systemic lupus erythematosus cardiomyopathy secondary to severe arrhythmia or volume overload, dilatative cardiomyopathy myocardial impairment in severe fetal growth restriction endocardial fibroelastosis of the right ventricle

REFERENCES

1. DeVore GR, Horenstein J, Siassi B, Lawrence DP. Fetal echocardiography. VII. Doppler color flow mapping: a new technique for the diagnosis of congenital heart disease. *Am J Obstet Gynecol* 1987;156:1054–64

2. Gembruch U, Hansmann M, Redel D, Bald R. Fetal two-dimensional Doppler echocardiography (color flow mapping) and its place in prenatal diagnosis. *Prenat Diagn* 1989;9:535–47

3. Kurjak A, Breyer B, Jurkovic D, Alfirevic Z, Miljan M. Color flow mapping in obstetrics. *J Perinat Med* 1987;15:271–81

4. Chaoui R, Bollmann R. Fetal color Doppler echocardiography. 1. General principles and normal findings (German). *Ultraschall Med* 1994;15:100–4

5. Rice MJ, McDonald RW, Sahn DJ. Contributions of color Doppler to the evaluation of cardiovascular abnormalities in the fetus. *Semin Ultrasound CT MR* 1993;14:277–85

6. Chaoui R, Bollmann R. Fetal color Doppler echocardiography. 2. Abnormalities of the heart and great vessels (German). *Ultraschall Med* 1994;15:105–11

7. Copel JA, Morotti R, Hobbins JC, Kleinman CS. The antenatal diagnosis of congenital heart disease using fetal echocardiography: is color flow mapping necessary? *Obstet Gynecol* 1991;78:1–8

8. DeVore G. The use of color Doppler imaging to examine the fetal heart. Normal and pathologic anatomy. In Jaffe R, Warsof SL, eds. *Color Doppler Imaging in Obstetrics and Gynecology*. McGraw-Hill, 1992:121–54

9. Sharland G, Chita S, Allan L. The use of color Doppler in fetal echocardiography. *Int J Cardiol* 1990;28:229–36

10. Chiba Y, Kanzaki T, Kobayashi H, Murakami M, Yutani C. Evaluation of fetal structural heart disase using color flow mapping. *Ultrasound Med Biol* 1990;16:221–9

11. Chaoui R, Bollmann R, Goldner B, Heling KS, Tennstedt C. Fetal cardiomegaly: echocardiographic findings and outcome in 19 cases. *Fetal Diagn Ther* 1994;9:92–104

12. Chaoui R, Goldner B, Heling K-S, Bollmann R. Intracardiac Doppler flow velocities in marked fetal cardiomegaly. *J Matern Fetal Invest* 1995;5:68–73

13. Chaoui R, Tennstedt C, Goldner B, Bollmann R. Prenatal diagnosis of ventriculo-coronary communications in a second-trimester fetus using transvaginal and transabdominal color Doppler sonography. *Ultrasound Obstet Gynecol* 1997;9:194–7

14. Gembruch U, Chatterjee M, Bald R, Redel D, Hansmann M. Prenatal diagnosis of aortic atresia by colour Doppler flow mapping. *Prenat Diagn* 1990;10:211–15

15. Hata K, Hata T, Manabe A, Kitao M. Hypoplastic left heart syndrome: color Doppler sonographic and magnetic resonance imaging features in utero. *Gynecol Obstet Invest* 1995;39:70–2

16. Gembruch U, Knopfle G, Chatterjee M, Bald R, Redel DA, Fodisch HJ, Hansmann M. Prenatal diagnosis of atrioventricular canal malformations with up-to-date echocardiographic technology: report of 14 cases. *Am Heart J* 1991;121:1489–97

17. Respondek ML, Kammermeier M, Ludomirsky A, Weil SR, Huhta JC. The prevalence and clinical significance of fetal tricuspid valve regurgitation with normal heart anatomy. *Am J Obstet Gynecol* 1994;171:1265–70

18. Gembruch U, Smrcek JM. The prevalence and clinical significance of tricuspid valve regurgitation in normally grown fetuses and those with intrauterine growth retardation. *Ultrasound Obstet Gynecol* 1997;9:374–82

13

Color Doppler sonography in the diagnosis of fetal abnormalities

Rabih Chaoui

INTRODUCTION

Color Doppler plays a vital role in the diagnosis of fetal cardiac defects and in the assessment of the hemodynamic responses to fetal hypoxia and anemia. This chapter examines an additional role of color Doppler in the diagnosis of non-cardiac malformations. In the future, color Doppler may also be used in the three-dimensional reconstruction and visualization of fetal and placental vessels[1,2].

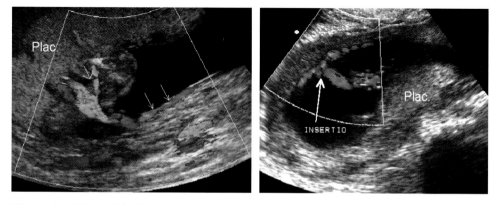

Figure 1 The umbilical cord inserts into an anterior placenta but an umbilical vessel extends into the amniotic membranes (left). In this fetus with a posterior placenta, there is velamentous insertion of the umbilical cord (right)

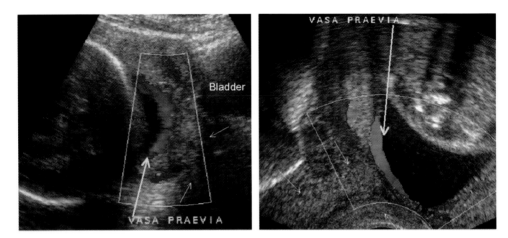

Figure 2 Transabdominal demonstration of a vasa previa in a fetus in vertex position (left). In this condition, transvaginal color Doppler sonography demonstrates the presence of fetal vessels within the membranes across the internal cervical os (right). The yellow arrows point to the vasa previa and the white arrows to the cervix

PLACENTAL AND UMBILICAL VESSELS

The umbilical cord vessels can be followed from their placental insertion (Figure 1) to their attachment on the fetal abdominal wall and their extension into the fetal abdomen[3]. Color Doppler is useful in the diagnosis of vasa previa (Figure 2), and targeted examination for this condition should always be undertaken in patients with velamentous insertion of the cord (Figure 1), succenturiate lobe, placenta previa, multiple gestation and amniotic bands[4–8]. Color Doppler is also helpful in the detection of placenta accreta[9,10] and chorioangioma, which is an arteriovenous fistulous malformation within the placenta[11,12].

Examination of the umbilical cord facilitates the detection of nuchal cord (Figure 3), false and true knots of the cord (Figure 3), hemangioma or angiomyxoma of the cord, hypoplastic umbilical artery, fusion of two arteries into one, and a single umbilical artery[13–21]. In a transverse view of the lower abdomen, the two umbilical arteries (superior vesical arteries) are seen on either side of the bladder (Figure 4) and, using this plane, it is easier to diagnose a single umbilical artery than by examining a cross-section of the umbilical cord.

A varix or aneurysm of the intra-abdominal part of the umbilical vein is recognized as a hypoechoic cyst and the diagnosis can be made by color Doppler (Figure 5)[22,23]. Color Doppler can also facilitate the diagnosis of an abnormal course of the umbilical vein, including a persistent right umbilical vein (Figures 6 and 7), and absence of the

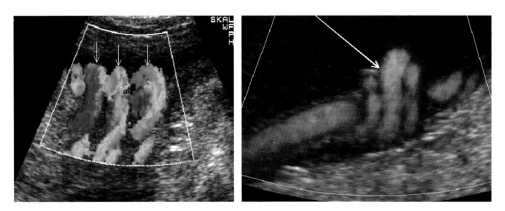

Figure 3 Three-fold nuchal cord (left). False knot of the umbilical cord (right)

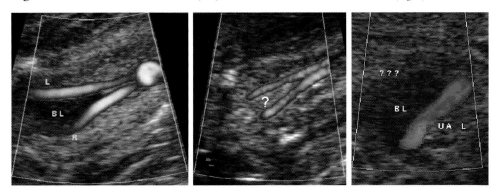

Figure 4 Transverse section of the fetal lower abdomen demonstrating the bladder and the umbilical arteries (left). In a fetus with Potter syndrome, there is no visible bladder (?) between the umbilical arteries (middle). In this fetus, there is only a single umbilical artery (right)

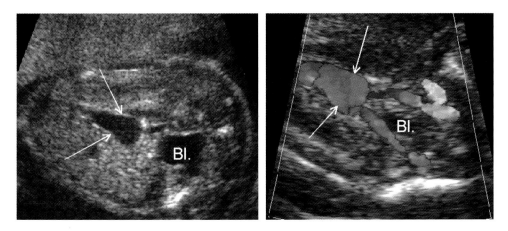

Figure 5 Transverse section of the fetal lower abdomen demonstrating two cystic structures (left). Color Doppler demonstrates that one cyst is the bladder with both umbilical arteries and the other cyst is a varix of the umbilical vein (right)

ductus venosus with direct connection of the umbilical vein to the right atrium (Figure 7), inferior vena cava or iliac vein[24–28]. In two fetuses with Down syndrome, we detected a fistula between the hepatic artery and the ductus venosus[29].

In monochorionic twins, color Doppler is useful in the identification of placental vascular communications in pregnancies with twin-to-twin transfusion syndrome, in the detection of retrograde perfusion in twin reversed arterial perfusion (TRAP) sequence and in the diagnosis of cord entanglement in monoamniotic twins[30,31].

RENAL VESSELS

Color Doppler examination of fetal renal vessels can facilitate the diagnosis of renal malformations. It is best to use a coronal view of the fetus, allowing visualization of the descending aorta with both the left and right renal arteries (Figure 8). Color Doppler is useful in the diagnosis of unilateral or bilateral renal agenesis (Figure 9), double arterial supply of a normal or a duplex kidney (Figure 8), horseshoe kidney (Figure 10) and pelvic kidney[32–38].

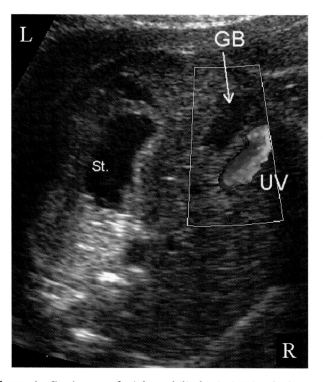

Figure 6 Persistence of a right umbilical vein (UV), which is seen to the right of the gallbladder (GB) and stomach (St.)

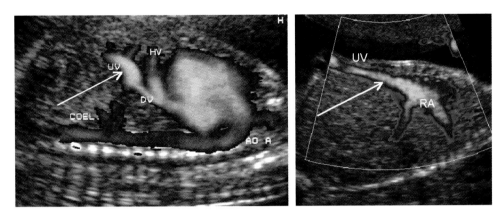

Figure 7 Longitudinal view of the fetal trunk and abdomen demonstrating the umbilical vein and ductus venosus in their course through the liver towards the heart (left). In this fetus with absence of the ductus venosus, the umbilical vein does not enter the liver and communicates directly with the right atrium (right)

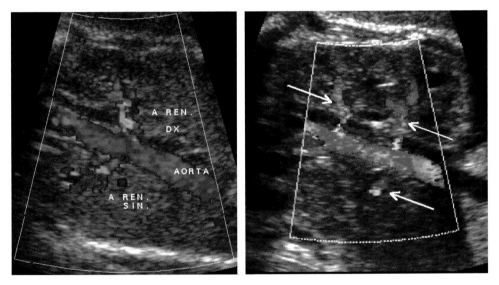

Figure 8 Coronal view of the descending aorta demonstrating both renal arteries (left). Duplex kidney with arterial supply by two renal vessels (right)

INTRACRANIAL VESSELS

Color Doppler is helpful in the diagnosis of intracranial arteriovenous fistulae, such as vein of Galen aneurym (Figure 11) and in distinguishing this vascular malformation from an arachnoid cyst, porencephaly or hydrocephaly[39–42]. Intracranial arteriovenous fistulae can be also found in other regions of the brain and do not always present as a

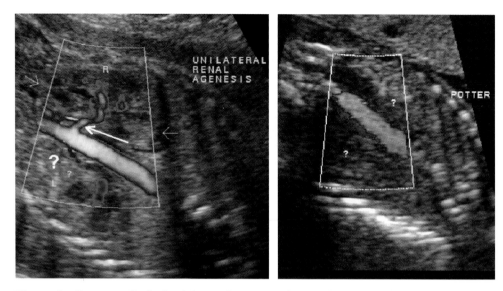

Figure 9 Presence of only the right renal artery in a fetus with agenesis of the left kidney (left). In a fetus with bilateral renal agenesis, there are no renal arteries arising from the aorta (right)

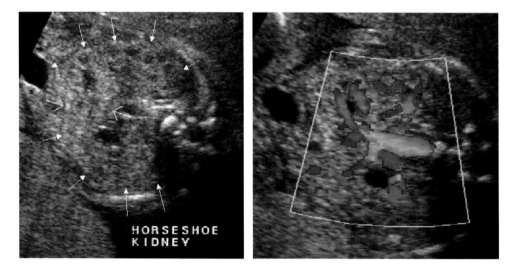

Figure 10 Horseshoe kidney diagnosed by real-time ultrasound (left) is confirmed by color Doppler (right)

hypoechoic cyst. In such cases, a fistula is suspected by the presence of the associated cardiomegaly and dilated neck veins, and the diagnosis is made by targeted examination of the brain with color Doppler. Some malformations of the fetal brain are often

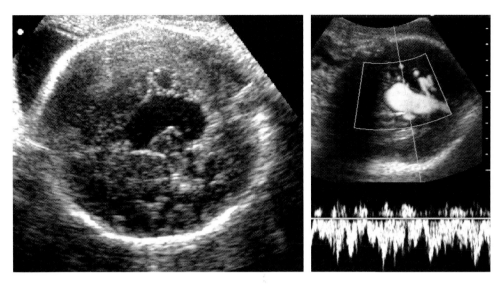

Figure 11 Vein of Galen aneurysm as an intracerebral cystic structure in gray scale (left) and as a vascular malformation with color Doppler (right)

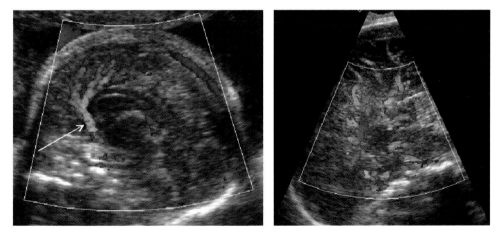

Figure 12 Midsagittal view of the head demonstrating the anterior (pericallosal) cerebral artery in a normal fetus (left). In a fetus with agenesis of the corpus callosum, there is abnormal looping and ramification of the pericallosal artery (right)

associated with an abnormal course of intracranial vessels and their visualization using color Doppler can be used for confirming the diagnosis. Agenesis or dysgenesis of the corpus callosum is associated with an abnormal looping of the pericallosal artery (Figure 12), and, in microcephaly and holoprosencephaly, the shape of the circle of Willis may be distorted (Figure 13)[43,44].

INTRATHORACIC VESSELS

Pulmonary arteries and veins can be seen in their course from the heart into the peripheral pulmonary segments, and Doppler measurements in these vessels may be useful in the detection of pulmonary hypoplasia[45–49]. In suspected diaphragmatic hernia, visualization of liver vessels in the thorax can confirm the diagnosis and has prognostic value[50,51]. Color Doppler has also been found to be useful in the diagnosis of the very rare condition of unilateral lung agenesis[52]. In bronchopulmonary

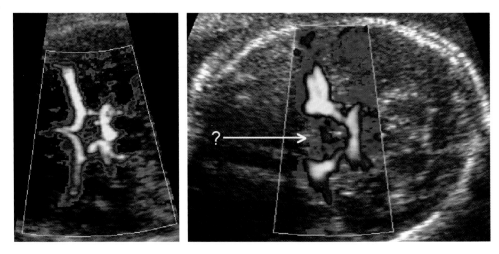

Figure 13 Circle of Willis in a normal fetus (left). In holoprosencephaly, the anterior artery is part of the malformation and the circle is not closed (right)

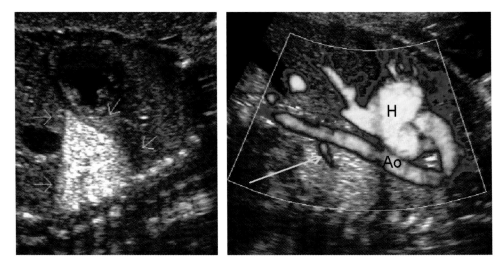

Figure 14 Pulmonary sequestration (left) with the feeding artery arising directly from the descending aorta (right)

sequestration, the diagnosis can be made by the demonstration of the feeding artery arising directly from the descending aorta (Figure 14)[53,54]. Some cardiac defects, such as pulmonary valve atresia with ventricular septum defect, are associated with multiple aorto-pulmonary collateral arteries which may complicate the neonatal course.

INTRA-ABDOMINAL VESSELS

Color Doppler has made it possible to visualize the celiac trunk with the hepatic, superior mesenteric, splenic, adrenal and other arteries. In general, the differential diagnosis of abdominal wall defects is easy by gray-scale imaging, but, in some cases, color Doppler may be necessary to demonstrate the attachment of the umbilical cord and to help distinguish between an omphalocele and a gastroschisis (Figure 15). However, in these conditions, Doppler measurements in the superior mesenteric artery have not been found to be useful in predicting postnatal outcome[55]. Color Doppler is useful in the diagnosis of hepatic hemangioma, aortic aneurysm, aneurysm of the umbilical vein (Figure 5), and infradiaphragmatic anomalous pulmonary venous drainage[56–58]. In fetuses with left isomerism (polysplenia), color Doppler can facilitate visualization of the dilated azygous vein near the descending aorta and confirmation of the absence of the inferior vena cava (Figure 16).

FETAL TUMORS

Fetal tumors are rare but, for optimal perinatal management, their differential diagnosis and precise description are desirable. In fetal goiter, color Doppler demonstrates high perfusion of the thyroid gland[59,60]. Echogenic or cystic lesions in the upper part of the

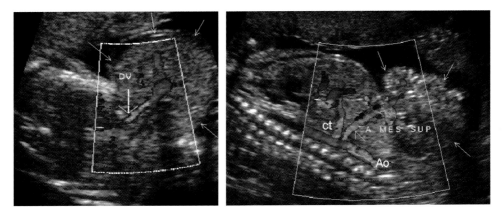

Figure 15 Umbilical vein and ductus venosus in a fetus with exomphalos (left). Gastroschisis with demonstration of the descending aorta, the celiac trunk (ct) and the superior mesenteric artery extending into the exteriorized bowel (right)

kidneys may represent a neuroblastoma, adrenal hemorrhage or congenital adrenal hypertrophy, and the differential diagnosis could be facilitated by visualization of the adrenal arteries by color Doppler[61,62]. Color Doppler is also useful in the distinction of sacrococcygeal teratoma, which is vascular (Figure 17), from other cystic lesions, such

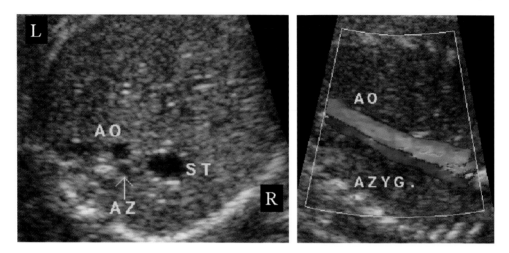

Figure 16 Fetus with left isomerism (polysplenia). A cross-section in the upper abdomen shows the stomach (ST) on the right side, no inferior vena cava and the dilated azygous vein near the aorta (left). In the longitudinal coronal view, different flow directions in the aorta and in the azygous vein are demonstrated by color Doppler (right)

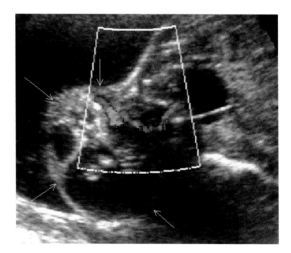

Figure 17 Vessels within a sacrococcygeal teratoma demonstrated by color Doppler

as meningocele or ectodermal cyst[63,64]. A teratoma can also be found in other sites, like the abdomen, thorax or neck. Color Doppler can be used in diagnosing lymphangioma and hemangioma but, in these conditions, flow velocities are very low[65–67].

VISUALIZATION OF FLUID MOVEMENTS

Color Doppler enables not only visualization of blood flow but also movement of fluid. During fetal breathing movements, flow can be observed at the level of the mouth, nose and trachea (Figure 18)[68–70]. Color Doppler facilitates the diagnosis of cleft palate by demonstrating the movement of fluid between mouth and nose during breathing movements[71,72]. In normal fetuses, there is movement of fluid in the trachea during breathing movements and the flow has been shown to be decreased in those fetuses with diaphragmatic hernia and lethal pulmonary hypoplasia, but not in those that survive[73]. In laryngeal atresia, there is no fluid flow within the dilated trachea[74].

In fetuses with duodenal stenosis or atresia, to-and-fro fluid movements can be observed within the stomach (Figure 19), which presumably represent abnormal peristaltic movements. The appearance of this sign may precede the development of the double-bubble sign and polyhydramnios[75]. Similarly, in fetuses with ureteric dilatation and peristalsis, color Doppler may be useful in the diagnosis of vesico-ureteric reflux. In fetuses with suspected genital abnormalities, visualization of urination by color Doppler may help to make the diagnosis of hypospadias.

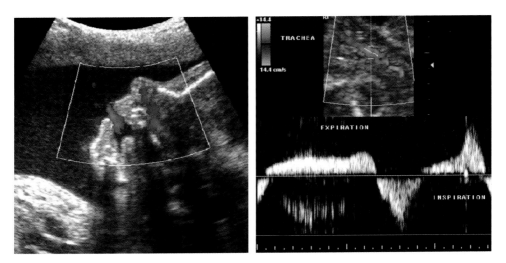

Figure 18 Breathing through the nose and mouth in a third-trimester fetus (left). Visualization of the trachea in color Doppler also demonstrates flow. Pulsed Doppler examination allows the demonstration of fluid flow movements during expiration and inspiration (right)

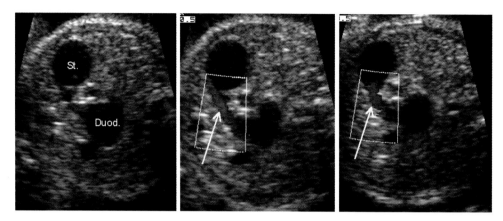

Figure 19 Duodenal atresia with the double-bubble sign of dilated stomach and proximal duodenum (left). Peristalsis and antiperistalsis waves are associated with to-and-fro fluid movements (red and blue) demonstrated by color Doppler (middle and right)

In fetuses treated with pleuro–amniotic or vesico–amniotic shunts, color Doppler may be useful in demonstrating patency of the shunts and continuing drainage of fluid from the fetus into the amniotic fluid.

DIFFERENTIAL DIAGNOSIS OF OLIGOHYDRAMNIOS

There are essentially three causes of absence or severe reduction in amniotic fluid at mid-pregnancy: premature rupture of the membranes, bilateral renal agenesis or dysplasia, and severe hypoxia with intrauterine growth restriction. Color Doppler is useful in distinguishing between oligohydramnios and anhydramnios, where all the translucent areas in the amniotic cavity are filled with loops of umbilical cord. In hypoxic growth restriction, the fetal measurements are small for gestation, the fetal heart looks dilated and the bowel is echogenic. Doppler demonstrates the presence of two renal arteries and absent or reversed end-diastolic frequencies in the umbilical arteries. In renal agenesis or dysplasia, umbilical artery Doppler is normal, but no renal vessels are seen (Figure 9) and no bladder filling is observed between the intra-abdominal umbilical arteries (Figure 4). In premature rupture of the membranes, there are normal renal vessels, normal umbilical flow and normal filling of the bladder.

REFERENCES

1. Chaoui R, Kalache K, Bollmann R. Three-dimensional color power angiography in the assessment of fetal vascular anatomy under normal and abnormal conditions. In Kupesic S, Kurjak A, eds. *Three-Dimensional Power Doppler in Obstetrics and Gynecology.* Carnforth, UK: Parthenon Publishing, 2000:150–8

2. Chaoui R, Kalache K. Three-dimensional color power imaging: principles and first experience in prenatal diagnosis. In Merz E, ed. *3D Ultrasonography in Obstetrics and Gynecology.* Philadelphia: Lippincott, Williams and Wilkins, 1998:135–42

3. Di Salvo DN, Benson CB, Laing FC, Brown DL, Frates MC, Doubilet PM. Sonographic evaluation of the placental cord insertion site. *Am J Roentgenol* 1998;170:1295–8

4. Raga F, Ballester MJ, Osborne NG, Bonilla Musoles F. Role of color flow Doppler ultrasonography in diagnosing velamentous insertion of the umbilical cord and vasa previa. A report of two cases. *J Reprod Med* 1995;40:804–8

5. Arts H, van Eyck J. Antenatal diagnosis of vasa previa by transvaginal color Doppler sonography. *Ultrasound Obstet Gynecol* 1993;3:276–8

6. Daly Jones E, Hollingsworth J, Sepulveda W. Vasa praevia: second trimester diagnosis using colour flow imaging. *Br J Obstet Gynaecol* 1996;103:284–6

7. Meyer WJ, Blumenthal L, Cadkin A, Gauthier DW, Rotmensch S. Vasa previa: prenatal diagnosis with transvaginal color Doppler flow imaging. *Am J Obstet Gynecol* 1993;169:1627–9

8. Oyelese KO, Schwarzler P, Coates S, Sanusi FA, Hamid R, Campbell S. A strategy for reducing the mortality rate from vasa previa using transvaginal sonography with color Doppler. *Ultrasound Obstet Gynecol* 1998;12:434–8

9. Chou MM, Ho ESC, Lu F, Lee YH. Prenatal diagnosis of placenta previa/accreta with color Doppler ultrasound. *Ultrasound Obstet Gynecol* 1992;2:293–6

10. Lerner JP, Deane S, Timor-Tritsch IE. Characterization of placenta accreta using transvaginal sonography and color Doppler imaging. *Ultrasound Obstet Gynecol* 1995;5:198–201

11. Zoppini C, Acaia B, Lucci G, Pugni L, Tassis B, Nicolini U. Varying clinical course of large placental chorioangiomas. Report of 3 cases. *Fetal Diagn Ther* 1997;12:61–4

12. D'Ercole C, Cravello L, Boubli L, Labit C, Millet V, Potier A, Blanc B. Large chorioangioma associated with hydrops fetalis: prenatal diagnosis and management. *Fetal Diagn Ther* 1996;11:357–60

13. Pilu G, Falco P, Guazzarini M, Sandri F, Bovicelli L. Sonographic demonstration of nuchal cord and abnormal umbilical artery waveform heralding fetal distress. *Ultrasound Obstet Gynecol* 1998;12:125–7

14. Jauniaux E, Mawissa C, Peellaerts C, Rodesch F. Nuchal cord in normal third-trimester pregnancy: a color Doppler imaging study. *Ultrasound Obstet Gynecol* 1992;2:417–19

15. Sepulveda W, Shennan AH, Bower S, Nicolaidis P, Fisk NM. True knot of the umbilical cord: a difficult prenatal ultrasonographic diagnosis. *Ultrasound Obstet Gynecol* 1995;5:106–8

16. Gembruch U, Baschat AA. True knot of the umbilical cord: transient constrictive effect to umbilical venous blood flow demonstrated by Doppler sonography. *Ultrasound Obstet Gynecol* 1996;8:53–6

17. Tennstedt C, Chaoui R, Bollmann R, Dietel M. Angiomyxoma of the umbilical cord in one twin with cystic degeneration of Wharton's jelly. A case report. *Pathol Res Pract* 1998;194:55–8

18. Sepulveda W, Flack NJ, Bower S, Fisk NM. The value of color Doppler ultrasound in the prenatal diagnosis of hypoplastic umbilical artery. *Ultrasound Obstet Gynecol* 1994;4:143–6

19. Persutte WH, Hobbins J. Single umbilical artery: a clinical enigma in modern prenatal diagnosis. *Ultrasound Obstet Gynecol* 1995;6:216–29

20. Abuhamad AZ, Shaffer W, Mari G, Copel JA, Hobbins JC, Evans AT. Single umbilical artery: does it matter which artery is missing? *Am J Obstet Gynecol* 1995;173:728–32

21. Jauniaux E. The single artery umbilical cord: it is worth screening for antenatally? *Ultrasound Obstet Gynecol* 1995;5:75–6

22. Sepulveda W, Mackenna A, Sanchez J, Corral E, Carstens E. Fetal prognosis in varix of the intrafetal umbilical vein. *J Ultrasound Med* 1998;17:171–5

23. Rizzo G, Arduini D. Prenatal diagnosis of an intra-abdominal ectasia of the umbilical vein with color Doppler ultrasonography. *Ultrasound Obstet Gynecol* 1992;2:55–7

24. Hill LM, Mills A, Peterson C, Boyles D. Persistent right umbilical vein: sonographic detection and subsequent neonatal outcome. *Obstet Gynecol* 1994;84:923–5

25. Chaoui R, Göldner B, Bollmann R. Prenatal diagnosis of two cases with absence of the ductus venosus associated with an atypical course of the umbilical vein: implications for the possible role of the ductus venosus. *Ultrasound Obstet Gynecol* 1994;4:179

26. Ariyuki Y, Hata T, Manabe A, Hata K, Kitao M. Antenatal diagnosis of persistent right umbilical vein. *J Clin Ultrasound* 1995;23:324–6

27. Moore L, Toi A, Chitayat D. Abnormalities of the intra-abdominal fetal umbilical vein: reports of four cases and a review of the literature. *Ultrasound Obstet Gynecol* 1996;7:21–5

28. Hartung J, Chaoui R, Kalache K, Heling KS, Bollmann R. Abnormalities of the fetal umbilical vein: prenatal diagnosis and fetal outcome. *Ultrasound Obstet Gynecol* 1998;12:52

29. Hartung J, Chaoui R, Tennstedt C, Bollmann R. Prenatal diagnosis of an intrahepatic arterio-venous fistula associated with Down syndrome: a report of two cases. *Ultrasound Obstet Gynecol* 2000;15:in press

30. Hecher K, Ville Y, Nicolaides KH. Color Doppler ultrasonography in the identification of communicating vessels in twin–twin transfusion syndrome and acardiac twins. *J Ultrasound Med* 1995;14:37–40

31. Schwarzler P, Ville Y, Moscoso G, Tennstedt C, Bollmann R, Chaoui R. Diagnosis of twin reversed arterial perfusion sequence in the first trimester by transvaginal color Doppler ultrasound. *Ultrasound Obstet Gynecol* 1999;13:143–6

32. Mackenzie FM, Kingston GO, Oppenheimer L. The early prenatal diagnosis of bilateral renal agenesis using transvaginal sonography and color Doppler ultrasonography. *J Ultrasound Med* 1994;13:49–51

33. Sepulveda W, Stagiannis KD, Flack NJ, Fisk NM. Accuracy of prenatal diagnosis of renal agenesis with color flow imaging in severe second-trimester oligohydramnios. *Am J Obstet Gynecol* 1995;173:1788–92

34. DeVore GR. The value of color Doppler sonography in the diagnosis of renal agenesis. *J Ultrasound Med* 1995;14:443–9

35. Sepulveda W, Romero R, Pryde PG, Wolfe HM, Addis JR, Cotton DB. Prenatal diagnosis of sirenomelus with color Doppler ultrasonography. *Am J Obstet Gynecol* 1994;170:1377–9

36. King KL, Kofinas AD, Simon NV, Clay D. Antenatal ultrasound diagnosis of fetal horseshoe kidney. *J Ultrasound Med* 1991;10:643–4

37. Hill LM, Grzybek P, Mills A, Hogge WA. Antenatal diagnosis of fetal pelvic kidney. *Obstet Gynecol* 1994;83:333–6

38. Meizner I, Yitzhak M, Levi A, Barki Y, Barnhard Y, Glezerman M. Fetal pelvic kidney: a challenge in prenatal diagnosis? *Ultrasound Obstet Gynecol* 1995;5:391–3

39. Dan U, Shalev E, Greif M, Weiner E. Prenatal diagnosis of fetal brain arteriovenous malformation: the use of color Doppler imaging. *J Clin Ultrasound* 1992;20:149–51

40. Paladini D, Palmieri S, D'Angelo A, Martinelli P. Prenatal ultrasound diagnosis of cerebral arteriovenous fistula. *Obstet Gynecol* 1996;88:678–81

41. Sepulveda W, Platt CC, Fisk NM. Prenatal diagnosis of cerebral arteriovenous malformation using color Doppler ultrasonography: case report and review of the literature. *Ultrasound Obstet Gynecol* 1995;6:282–6

42. Heling KS, Chaoui R, Bollmann R. Prenatal diagnosis of a Galen vein aneurysm using color Doppler and 3D power Doppler. *Ultrasound Obstet Gynecol* 2000;15:in press

43. Guzman ER, Walters C, Sharma S, Tierney R, Palermo A, Vintzileos AM. Two-dimensional gray-scale imaging and color Doppler in the detection of the corpus callosum and pericallosal artery. *Ultrasound Obstet Gynecol* 1999;14:53

44. Pilu G, Falco P, Milano V, Perolo A, Bovicelli L. Prenatal diagnosis of microcephaly assisted by vaginal sonography and power Doppler. *Ultrasound Obstet Gynecol* 1998;11:357–60

45. Rasanen J, Huhta JC, Weiner S, Wood DC, Ludomirski A. Fetal branch pulmonary arterial vascular impedance during the second half of pregnancy. *Am J Obstet Gynecol* 1996;174:1441–9

46. Chaoui R, Taddei F, Rizzo G, Bast C, Lenz F, Bollmann R. Doppler echocardiography of the main stems of the pulmonary arteries in the normal human fetus. *Ultrasound Obstet Gynecol* 1998;11:173–9

47. Roth P, Agnani G, Arbez Gindre F, Pauchard JY, Burguet A, Schaal JP, Maillet R. Use of energy color Doppler in visualizing fetal pulmonary vascularization to predict the absence of severe pulmonary hypoplasia. *Gynecol Obstet Invest* 1998;46:153–7

48. Chaoui R, Kalache K, Tennstedt C, Lenz F, Vogel M. Pulmonary arterial Doppler in fetuses with lung hypoplasia. *Eur J Obstet Gynecol Reprod Biol* 1999:84:179–85

49. Yoshimura S, Masuzaki H, Miura K, Muta K, Gotoh H, Ishimaru T. Diagnosis of fetal pulmonary hypoplasia by measurement of blood flow velocity waveforms of pulmonary arteries with Doppler ultrasonography. *Am J Obstet Gynecol* 1999;180:441–6

50. Sherer DM, Eglinton GS, Goncalves LF, Lewis KM, Queenan JT. Prenatal color and pulsed Doppler sonographic documentation of intrathoracic umbilical vein and ductus venosus, confirming extensive hepatic herniation in left congenital diaphragmatic hernia. *Am J Perinatol* 1996;13:159–62

51. Botash RJ, Spirt BA. Color Doppler imaging aids in the prenatal diagnosis of congenital diaphragmatic hernia. *J Ultrasound Med* 1993;12:359–61

52. Kalache KD, Chaoui R, Paris S, Bollmann R. Prenatal diagnosis of right lung agenesis using color Doppler and magnetic resonance imaging. *Fetal Diagn Ther* 1997;12:360–2

53. Morin L, Crombleholme TM, Louis F, D'Alton ME. Bronchopulmonary sequestration: prenatal diagnosis with clinicopathologic correlation. *Curr Opin Obstet Gynecol* 1994;6:479–81

54. Smulian JC, Guzman ER, Ranzini AC, Benito CW, Vintzileos AM. Color and duplex Doppler sonographic investigation of in utero spontaneous regression of pulmonary sequestration. *J Ultrasound Med* 1996;15:789–92

55. Abuhamad AZ, Mari G, Cortina RM, Croitoru DP, Evans AT. Superior mesenteric artery Doppler velocimetry and ultrasonographic assessment of fetal bowel in gastroschisis: a prospective longitudinal study. *Am J Obstet Gynecol* 1997;176:985–90

56. Mejides AA, Adra AM, O'Sullivan MJ, Nicholas MC. Prenatal diagnosis and therapy for a fetal hepatic vascular malformation. *Obstet Gynecol* 1995;85:850–3

57. Abuhamad AZ, Lewis D, Inati MN, Johnson DR, Copel JA. The use of color flow Doppler in the diagnosis of the fetal hepatic hemangioma. *J Ultrasound Med* 1993;4:223–6

58. DiSessa TG, Emerson DS, Felker RE, Brown DL, Cartier MS, Becker JA. Anomalous systemic and pulmonary venous pathways diagnosed in utero by ultrasound. *J Ultrasound Med* 1990;9:311–17

59. Soliman S, McGrath F, Brennan B, Glazebrook K. Color Doppler imaging of the thyroid gland in a fetus with congenital goiter: a case report. *Am J Perinatol* 1994;11:21–3

60. Luton D, Fried D, Sibony O, Vuillard E, Tebeka B, Boissinot C, Leger J, Polak M, Oury JF, Blot P. Assessment of fetal thyroid function by colored Doppler echography. *Fetal Diagn Ther* 1997;12: 24–7

61. Schwarzler P, Bernard JP, Senat MV, Ville Y. Prenatal diagnosis of fetal adrenal masses: differentiation between hemorrhage and solid tumor by color Doppler sonography. *Ultrasound Obstet Gynecol* 1999;13:351–5

62. Goldstein I, Gomez K, Copel JA. The real-time and color Doppler appearance of adrenal neuroblastoma in a third-trimester fetus. *Obstet Gynecol* 1994;83:854–6

63. Sherer DM, Fromberg RA, Rindfusz DW, Harris BH, Sanz LE. Color Doppler aided prenatal diagnosis of a type 1 cystic sacrococcygeal teratoma simulating a meningomyelocele. *Am J Perinatol* 1997;14:13–15

64. Bloechle M, Bollmann R, Wit J, Buttenberg S, Kursawe R, Guski H. Neuroectodermal cyst may be a rare differential diagnosis of fetal sacrococcygeal teratoma: first case report of a prenatally observed neuroectodermal cyst. *Ultrasound Obstet Gynecol* 1996;7:64–7

65. Bulas DI, Johnson D, Allen JF, Kapur S. Fetal hemangioma – sonographic and color flow Doppler findings. *J Ultrasound Med* 1992;11:499–501

66. Goncalves LF, Pereira ET, Parente LM, Vitorello DA, Barbosa UC, Saab Neto JA. Cutaneous hemangioma of the thigh: prenatal diagnosis. *Ultrasound Obstet Gynecol* 1997;9:128–30

67. Raman S, Ramanujam T, Lim CT. Prenatal diagnosis of an extensive haemangioma of the fetal leg: a case report. *J Obstet Gynaecol Res* 1996; 22:375–8

68. Bruner JP, Coggins T. Assessment of fetal breathing movements using three different ultrasound modalities. *J Clin Ultrasound* 1995;23:551–3

69. Suzuki M, Saito H, Yanaihara T. Assessment of fetal nasal fluid flow by two-dimensional color Doppler ultrasonography during pregnancy. *J Matern Fetal Med* 1999;8:159–63

70. Kalache KD, Chaoui R, Bollmann R. Doppler assessment of tracheal and nasal fluid flow during fetal breathing movements: preliminary observations. *Ultrasound Obstet Gynecol* 1997;9:257–61

71. Aubry M-C, Aubry J-P. Prenatal diagnosis of cleft palate: contribution of color Doppler ultrasound. *Ultrasound Obstet Gynecol* 1992;2:221–4

72. Monni G, Ibba RM, Olla G, Cao A, Crisponi G. Color Doppler ultrasound and prenatal diagnosis of cleft palate. *J Clin Ultrasound* 1995;23:189–91

73. Kalache KD, Chaoui R, Hartung J, Wernecke KD, Bollmann R. Doppler assessment of tracheal fluid flow during fetal breathing movements in cases of congenital diaphragmatic hernia. *Ultrasound Obstet Gynecol* 1998;12:27–32

74. Kalache KD, Chaoui R, Tennstedt C, Bollmann R. Prenatal diagnosis of laryngeal atresia in two cases of congenital high airway obstruction syndrome (CHAOS). *Prenat Diagn* 1997;17:577–81

75. Rizzo G, Capponi A, Arduini D, Romanini C. Prenatal diagnosis of gastroesophageal reflux by color and pulsed Doppler ultrasonography in a case of congenital pyloric atresia. *Ultrasound Obstet Gynecol* 1995; 6:290–2

Index